Riding with Miss Lindsey

Millennial Mind Publishing
An imprint of American Book Publishing
P.O. Box 65624
Salt Lake City, UT 84165
www.american-book.com
Printed in the United States of America on acid-free paper.
Riding with Miss Lindsey
Designed by Lucinda Vessey, design@american-book.com

Publisher's Note: *American Book Publishing relies on the author's integrity of research and attribution; each statement has not been investigated to determine if it has been accurately made. The author and publisher specifically disclaim any responsibility for any liability, loss, or risk, personal or otherwise, which is incurred as a consequence, directly or indirectly, of the use and application of any of the contents of this book. In such situations where medical, legal, or other professional services may apply, please seek the advice of such professionals directly.*

ISBN 1-58982-359-1
Library of Congress Cataloging-in-Publication Data
Alexander, Jim, 1960-
 Riding with Miss Lindsey / Jim Alexander.
     p. cm.
 Includes bibliographical references and index.
 ISBN 1-58982-359-1 (alk. paper)
 1. Alexander, Lindsey Michelle, 1987-2003--Health. 2. Down syndrome--Patients--
Biography. 3. Congenital heart disease in children--Surgery. I. Title.
 RJ506.D8A44 2006
 362.196'8588420092--dc22
 [B]
                        2006012944

Special Sales

These books are available at special discounts for bulk purchases. Special editions, including personalized covers, excerpts of existing books, and corporate imprints, can be created in large quantities for special needs. For more information e-mail
info@american-book.com.

Riding with Miss Lindsey

Jim Alexander

Dedicated to my little buttercup, who never gave up on anything.

Foreword

I met Lindsey and her parents, Jim and Donna, on the day of Lindsey's birth; journeyed with them episodically throughout her life and illness; and shared their grief at her death. When I first met her, the impact of her life on mine was unknowable. I had just arrived from California, having completed my formal training in caring for children with congenital heart disease. Little did I know that my real learning was about to begin, and Lindsey and her parents would be my teachers. Of course, I learned the obvious medical lessons available to all physicians who are attentive to their patients. But upon reflection I find that Lindsey and her parents taught me so much more about growing and developing our human potential in the face of adversity.

Lindsey's heart disease was life-threatening from the start, and survival was an ongoing challenge. Each new setback or noxious medical intervention was a test of character. By nature, some children shrink from these challenges; others show unfathomable courage. Lindsey summoned her strong will, became an active participant in reaching her therapeutic goals, and repeatedly passed the test.

Lindsey's difficult medical journey also teaches that suffering through hardships can have positive value, yielding toughness, maturity, and nobility of character not otherwise realized. Persistently enduring downturns in her condition, particularly when the outcome was uncertain, followed by improvement and recovery resulted in feelings of accomplishment against the odds and renewed optimism.

Lindsey and her parents also taught me that hope is an essential ingredient in sustaining life and health. Lindsey's heart and lungs did not read the same medical textbooks that I did, and often did not respond to treatment as expected. In counseling her parents, I tried to be realistic but not as outright pessimistic as I sometimes felt. In their wisdom, Lindsey's parents maintained a dogged, hopeful optimism, facing each new obstacle with the expectation of success. More often than not, they were right, I was wrong, and Lindsey improved.

Lindsey's compromised health presented many special needs and placed additional demands on her family when compared to a family with healthy children. I imagine that Jim and Donna would have given anything for Lindsey's heart disease to be easily and permanently fixed at birth. But in a way, the extra effort and additional requirements that Lindsey's needs demanded were a gift that deepened the family bond and broadened the circle of family and friends who participated in her care and were blessed by their involvement.

Foreword

For a busy physician caring for children with complex life-threatening conditions to remain detached and to not reflect on the impact of the chronic illness and death of a child on loved ones is sometimes excused as self-preservation. But for a physician to do so is to lose an opportunity to acknowledge and participate in the grief and loss of a child, and to miss learning lessons about the strength of character of the survivors. Modern medicine seeks to heal and prolong life and to measure success in years of life added, but the influence of a short life can be profound. It is not the years in your life but the life in your years that is the proper measure. Lindsey and her parents have taught me these and other lessons not learned in medical school, and for this I am grateful.

Elman Frantz, M.D.
Chapel Hill, North Carolina

Preface

The sun shimmered on the lake this fine spring morning. I thought about how lucky I was to have had a morning traveling partner all those years and having been able to see the lake together. I thought about how something experienced alone is never as special as when you see it through someone else's eyes. In just a few fleeting moments I was across the bridge and the beautiful view was gone. In a way, I reasoned, this was like Lindsey's life—a short span of sixteen years that we crossed like a bridge over a lake with a fabulous view. Then it was gone and we were left with lots of memories, pictures, videos, and a world of grief.

Being around Lindsey was like wearing special glasses because she pulled you into her world. When she passed, I realized those "Lindsey glasses" were taken away, and I thought to myself, "You know, that world was a pretty cool place." It was full of joy, humor, and excitement about the next thing to do or even something as simple as the next meal. I think I want to find those glasses again someday and put them on forever.

More than just grief is my motivation for writing. It is a need to preserve that memory the way I felt it, kind of like laminating an important document. I fear the passing of time will dull that, too. My lesson learned is that love for someone other than yourself is the only thing that really matters in this world. You can make yourself believe whatever you want, but what Lindsey taught us is that love cannot be dulled, medicated, or taken away.

If one could say greatness is what you do with what God gave you, then my daughter Lindsey achieved as much as a novice scaling the 14,000-foot Mount Lindsey in Colorado. Some people were lulled into believing that she was really just an ordinary kid five years younger than she really was—someone who was sometimes a little stubborn and sluggish. In these cases those folks did not have a clue about the underlying things going on with her physically, which was actually a compliment. Sometimes it took people a little while to realize Lindsey had Down syndrome. I laughed when someone who talked to her when she answered the phone told me later they did not realize there was anything different about her. Her speech continued to improve as she matured.

Along with Down syndrome, Lindsey had a heart so defective that even some of the most seasoned pediatric cardiologists in the world could not figure out exactly how she worked and why she functioned at all. After many corrective surgeries early on she had managed to not only survive, but to thrive. When she looked good and felt good, which was often, people just never realized what was going on.

Lindsey had to take seven different types of medicine twice a day every day to keep her heart functioning well. Somehow she was blessed with a great appetite for healthy food, a sense of humor, and the ability to sleep ten hours every night. I believe this is what kept her going, along with her inner drive. It was as though God gave Lindsey a one-day Flex pass each day to get her by without her heart failing, and she took full advantage of it.

It was Lindsey's drive to participate and to overcome her physical limitations that put her into this level of acceptance in the first place. On occasion she could even promote jealousy among other girls her own age because of the attention she tended to get from men. It was as though they were annoyed that someone like her could attract attention away from them.

Most people simply fell in love with her because they got to know the person inside that went with the laugh, smile, and funny noises she often made. For me that happened the first time I held her, a few seconds after she was born, even though she could not smile or laugh yet. Once locked on, Lindsey never let people go; she would always joke and kid with them every time she saw them thereafter. She wasn't always good or always happy; in fact, she could be downright belligerent if folks weren't toeing the line for her. But even that part of her personality is greatly missed.

In a way Lindsey even fooled us, her own family, into thinking she would somehow eventually conquer her heart defects. After all, she had proven the doctors wrong so many times that we just figured she was going to be around for a long time, maybe even longer than her mother and I. Underneath I knew differently, but refused to divorce my optimism for her. Lindsey's body was growing and every function growing stronger—except for her heart, which was the renegade body part. Right up until the morning we drove to the hospital, paper airplanes were constructed, puzzles worked, meals consumed, and shopping notes were written.

In this little four-and-a-half-foot person I found joy in the purest sense I have ever known. That is why I am writing this now. I hope this book inspires other parents raising children with special needs who already know what I am saying, and that it inspires others to begin to know.

Chapter 1
The Early Days and Hospital Excursions

My wife, Donna, and I actually lost our first child to a miscarriage. The reason for the loss was unknown, and Donna put much effort into taking care of herself during her second pregnancy. Everything proceeded normally from the ultrasound through all checkups. Once, when Donna had some tea at lunch, the baby did some extra kicking that evening after supper.

We knew from the ultrasound that it was to be a baby girl, so we came up with the name Lindsey. Actually, my grandmother's maiden name was Lindsay, and one of my favorite uncles was named Lindsay. We liked the name, so we just changed the "a" to an "e." For a middle name we chose Michelle just because we liked the sound of it. From then on, the little bundle of energy in Donna's tummy was talked to as Lindsey Michelle Alexander or just "Lindsey."

Being the youngest in both of our families, Donna and I had very little notion of how to take care of a baby. We had no preconceived ideas of how a little baby was supposed to look or act. We knew this was going to be a life-altering education for us. Little did we know how much of an education was coming.

Of course I did the typical first-time father thing: I did not gas up the car prior to the labor coming on. We actually had to stop and fill up on the way to the hospital. I was a little nervous, but not too bad. Lindsey was ready to see us, and we were ready to see her, too.

We got checked into the hospital OK and proceeded to the birthing room. I stayed in the room with Donna. I did not realize how hard this process was for women, but felt better being there versus being outside.

The labor went pretty well. We had actually gone to classes, so we did the breathing exercises and I helped rub Donna's back. Donna had a natural childbirth this time, taking no medications. This may have been a blessing. Lindsey was born after about eight hours. She cried immediately, just like any other newborn, and I remember her scores being 8.5 out of 10. All looked well. Appearance-wise she looked like any other newborn baby, but having never really seen one I would not have known the difference. I got to hold her after a few seconds when they cut the cord. Of course I bonded with her right then.

It is hard to recollect everything after that, except I remember being in the hospital room with my wife and the nurse bringing in Lindsey for us to hold. For about thirty minutes we were as happy as any family can be. We suspected nothing. Then the nurse returned and said that they needed to get Lindsey back into the nursery to warm up, and we kissed her good-bye for a while.

Soon a pediatrician named Dr. Scott McGeary popped into the room. He told us that he wasn't sure, but he thought he may have noticed some characteristics of Down syndrome in Lindsey and they needed to test for it. The results would be known in about a week. He said that she did not have the classic features such as the heavy skin at the eyes or the hand markings, but he saw something.

Of course this immediately hit us right in the gut, but this was no fault of Dr. McGeary; he was very nice. We were totally unprepared and became very distraught. More unsettling news was to follow.

The doctor came back after a short time and reported some other revelations. He had noticed that Lindsey's coloration was not quite the same as other babies who are adapting to lung breathing versus what they do in the womb. He was also detecting some significant heart murmurs. He began taking blood samples to check the oxygen and carbon dioxide content. Dr. McGeary was amused and impressed with Lindsey and how she was so "feisty" when he drew blood.

On Lindsey's second day in the world, she rode in an ambulance to the University of North Carolina at Chapel Hill (UNC) Hospital to see a team of pediatric cardiologists. Donna walked herself into the hospital even though she was still in physical pain. This was to be our first trip of many to that hospital over the next few years.

I remember that when we hit the seventh-floor wing where most sick babies went, we saw a doctor smiling and just playing with a baby on a table. As we got closer we saw that this was our baby, Lindsey, and she was grabbing the finger of Dr. Elman Frantz. For some strange reason, everything was relaxed and non-chaotic at this point. Dr. Frantz had just come from UCLA to join the staff at UNC. Elman had a very calm demeanor and he was able to tell us right then what was wrong with Lindsey because they had done an ultrasound. The defect was called a "tetralogy of Fallot," which sounded to me more like a work of Shakespeare than a health problem. However, it is a severe heart defect in which multiple holes exist in the walls between the atria and the ventricles; the blood even can sometimes flow the wrong way.

There was also some pulmonary narrowing and restriction to her lungs. After we absorbed all that information, Dr. Frantz added that the outlook was far from hopeless; through a series of surgeries, sometimes the condition could be repaired enough for the patient to live many years. He told us that they would probably do a BT shunt surgery in about six weeks that would carry her to about one-and-a-half years old. Then they would need to do open-heart surgery to try to patch the holes and remove the obstruction. They wanted to do a heart catheterization in about three weeks in order to further determine the true extent of her defects. Elman was definitely sent to the right place at the right time, for there were many times over the years I felt that his judgment made a big difference. We remain grateful for that.

Surprisingly, we got to take Lindsey home after that. We did all the things new parents do. I do not believe she had to take a single medicine at that time. We changed diapers, and Lindsey actually got Mom's milk instead of formula by using a pump. We found out that even in her condition, this girl had a good appetite. She also slept just like any other baby. When she got upset, however, her color was sometimes blue-looking. This scared us a little. The good thing was that we had nothing to compare her to since neither of us had been around a baby before. We usually just sang to her and rocked her in my grandmother's old rocker. A few times at night I took her outside in the night air on the deck, since it was warm. For some reason, that always calmed her down. We even took her on a camping trip with her grandparents.

I could tell that Down syndrome was doing absolutely nothing to diminish what this child was about. We loved her and enjoyed being around her, and so did her grandparents. She seemed very alert to us, watching everything when she was awake. Donna decided she was not going back to work for a couple of years so she could stay home with her.

After a few weeks we brought Lindsey in for her heart catheterization. The risks were explained, but we felt they were pretty low, so we were not excessively worried. After they took her for the procedure and then a good bit of waiting, several doctors appeared with news that things were not going well at all. We were told that they would have to operate immediately or there would be no chance to save her. Any parent who has endured this type of waiting knows that it creates mind-wrecking anxiety. The doctors came back after about two hours and stated that she had survived and they had installed a BT shunt. They expected her to recover and do well for about a year or so, and then would require her first open-heart surgery.

After a week or so inside the intensive care unit, Lindsey came back to the seventh floor. Donna stayed with her full time once that happened. Lindsey got stronger, and they let us take her home after about another week. After that, we gained some sense of relief and felt more relaxed.

Lindsey was not on any medication during this period. She ate very well, slept well, and even got a little chubby. This continued for about eighteen months. I remember Lindsey's first birthday in her little yellow dress and the one candle on the cake. We have a picture of her giggling as I kissed her on the back of the neck with the single candle lit on the cake. We saw her personality coming out, and it was the dancing eyes of mischief and happiness I loved the most.

Lindsey's first open-heart surgery was a big event for us. This was Lindsey's first encounter with "Doc" Wilcox, a pretty famous pediatric heart surgeon at UNC. Dr. Frantz, Dr. Henry, and other pediatric cardiologists were also there to advise us of what to expect.

The surgery waiting room is a place of high anxiety, prayer, dread, and relief in most cases. I will never forget when Doc came into the waiting room. He was a towering man who looked and acted like Matt Dillon. He must have been through this so many times that he knew what to do, because he very quickly flashed us a smile as he entered. This was like a push button wired to an anxiety relief valve for us.

Lindsey survived this big surgery. Because of the extent of her defects, they could only attack one of them this time and still have her survive it. The goal was to do one more surgery to repair the rest. They told us she should recover and do pretty well, although she would require diuretic and potassium supplements. In a couple of years she would hopefully be ready to have the final surgery.

It took Lindsey more than a week in the intensive care unit and several weeks on the seventh floor to recover enough to come home. Donna would never leave Lindsey once she went to the seventh-floor unit. When they came home from the hospital, I constructed a large banner across our living room that said "WELCOME HOME LINDSEY AND DONNA."

Coming home from the hospital was always like starting a new life for the first time. It was like being given another chance at being together, and we were grateful that God had blessed us once again. When you have come so close to losing and fight so hard to survive, you see things differently. Working to own a mansion or a yacht becomes much less important than making smiles appear on a child's face.

To be honest, I cannot recall all of the details of the second or third heart surgeries. I remember that the second open-heart surgery happened as planned. The third surgery was a valve replacement, and Doc Wilcox was able to enlarge her pulmonary artery by splicing into it and sewing it. Doc Wilcox always used to visit Lindsey in the room prior to the surgery. He is coined a phrase during one of these visits that she never let go of: "You're a piece of work, Miss Lindsey." (She continued to say this to me and her mom even after she was sixteen years old. She would look at one of us and say, "You're a piece of work!") The last surgery turned out to be very successful in alleviating the pressure on the right side of Lindsey's heart. It was not enough to last a lifetime, but did enable many years of growth and happiness for all of us.

Recovery after surgery was never an easy path. I remember Donna staying with Lindsey at the hospital for one stretch of nine weeks straight. But Lindsey proved to always be a fighter who would not quit. She won every one of these early battles, thanks to God's grace guiding Doc, the pediatric cardiologists, and the intensive care nurses.

Donna and I were always lucky that others prayed for us and offered much support, particularly our employers, family members, and friends. Maggie Morris of UNC's cardiothoracic staff became a close friend of ours who always came in to brighten things up. Maggie always could make Lindsey smile and brought her things she could play with such as art and craft projects. Recovery and trips to the playroom were always considered good times instead of bad.

Each of these UNC surgeries was filled with the same stress, worry, hope, fear, and ultimate jubilation when we got to drive Miss Lindsey home one more time.

Lindsey's long-time pediatricians for checkups and hospital follow-ups were Dr. Lynne Wirth and Dr. Anita Martin, who were partners in the same office. Both doctors knew her well. Lindsey and Dr. Wirth had a unique relationship, because they usually saw each other only for checkups and more minor illnesses, so in general things were going fairly well during their visits. Lindsey loved to tease her, but Dr. Wirth told me later that Lindsey taught her how to slow down and to allow patients to do things on their own terms.

Lindsey called Dr. Wirth "Spaghetti and Meatballs"— for what reason, nobody knows. Once, Dr. Wirth got Lindsey good by showing up for a checkup appointment with a can of spaghetti and meatballs situated on her head. This brought out some raucous laughter from Lindsey.

Of course Lindsey was always a medical mystery, but Dr. Wirth and Dr. Martin certainly understood her well over the years and worked closely with her pediatric cardiologists at UNC.

Ironically, we still see Dr. Scott McGeary, Lindsey's original pediatrician, on occasion in an after-hours clinic he started. He even saw Lindsey on a few occasions after she was older. He always asked about her.

I cannot express enough gratitude for those who worked at Rex, Kaiser, Wake Med, and UNC hospitals. They took countless blood samples and X-rays and helped us through some very tough times with dignity and respect.

Chapter 2
Silly Girl with an Appetite for Fun

One thing we quickly learned was that Miss Lindsey was no wallflower. She loved to play and have a good time. I remember peeking at her through the rails of her crib and seeing a smile born that spread radiance like the sun breaking away from a summer cloud. My theory was that as long as Lindsey could smile, all was well in the world. My wife felt the same way, and the two of us put all we had into keeping things that way. Donna always had this lovable mischievous quality that transferred straight to Lindsey. Lindsey always loved to hide things, play practical jokes like tying your shoestrings together, or cover herself up with clothes in the laundry basket.

Lindsey had to sleep in a crib for much longer than most kids because she was slow to learn to stand and walk. But she could crawl, and it did not prevent her from doing many things.

Lindsey always gave the very best hugs. She grabbed you like a bear. In fact, Winnie the Pooh was one of Lindsey's favorite characters very early on. We bought her some of the early Disney videos, and we watched them over and over.

When Lindsey was around two years old, we used to sit on a bridge I built over a creek at our old home and play "Poohsticks." We would get two different sticks; one was mine and one was hers. The idea was for each of us to toss them into the water upstream at the same time. It was a race, and Lindsey loved the competition. We would say, "One, two, three, go!" and then toss the sticks and then spin to watch to see which stick would emerge from under the bridge first. Lindsey would giggle if her stick made it first and always wanted to do it again and again.

Lindsey was very sociable and knew no enemies, but I think a little of that is attributed to the positive aspects of Down syndrome. If people could just wear those Lindsey glasses for a while, then they would see the positive things in life instead of only the negative. Lindsey's viewpoint was to see joy in the simple things that many people take for granted. I never heard Lindsey state she was bored.

Lindsey's grandparents, aunts, and uncles definitely wore the glasses when she was around. She loved to go to visit them in Lexington, North Carolina. She brought them as much joy as anyone by just being there.

We found that Lindsey seemed to thrive the most when we took her places. She loved any festive place with lots of family, music, and chatter, and a party with all three was the ultimate to her. Food and laughter gave Lindsey an avenue for enjoying a life that otherwise would have been hard to travel.

We took her to buffet restaurants, and she developed an appetite for many different types of foods. She learned to like vegetables, fruits, meats, salads, and just about anything from any food group starting with her transition to solid food. When her baby teeth came in, Lindsey was better able to eat meats and harder-to-chew foods.

Salt was her one true enemy because of fluid retention, so we simply avoided salty foods. It really was never that hard. We all learned to do it. The fact is that most foods naturally have all the salt you need. When you don't add it, over time you learn to prefer not to have it. Lindsey made us all healthier in that respect.

At any restaurant, Lindsey loved to listen to the background music and watch other people while she was eating. She was strong enough to sit in a booster seat, so in general that was all she needed. We had to feed her for the first couple of years, but she caught on to feeding herself fairly quickly. She never was a particularly messy child (unlike her two later brothers) and seemed to be very neat when eating.

It took Lindsey a couple of years to start walking. Before that, she loved to climb up into a little plastic playhouse with a sliding board we had in our living room. She would go up and down it as many as twenty times in a row before tiring. Eventually she got strong enough to pull up, balance, and one day, *voilà*! She just took off. Once Lindsey started crawling, and especially when she started walking, we learned very quickly to safety-proof all of the kitchen cabinets and electrical outlets.

One thing Lindsey was good at during this time was throwing balls. She would do this very funny Popeye-type windup and then hurl a fireball back at you or somewhere else in the room.

Lindsey did not start talking very quickly. She definitely made many sounds, some of which imitated speech. She obviously had a lot to say, but as she grew older we could sense her frustration with not being able to speak. Early Intervention, a service funded by the state government, began working with her. Some of Lindsey's delay in speech was attributed to Down syndrome, but a lot of it was due to multiple ear infections. Down kids tend to have more underdeveloped Eustachian tubes, which do not drain properly during the early years of childhood. But Lindsey soon found a way to overcome this obstacle.

Chapter 3
Learning Sign Language, Starting School, and Special Olympics

A lady named Dee came once a week from Early Intervention to work with Lindsey and taught her sign language for many common but simple commands. Lindsey picked it up very quickly, and we could see the frustration that had been building in her just start to melt away like an ice cube on a warm sunny day. When she was thirsty or hungry, Lindsey could now tell us very quickly by signing. We got a book on signing so we could understand more of the signs and also teach Lindsey even more words. Lindsey began to identify things she saw outside or inside the house by signing. I especially remember her doing "tree" and "squirrel" when she was sitting at the table looking out the sliding-glass door.

I remember one of her favorite early books was one with a little boy going to the airport and getting a tour of an airplane. She used to do the sign for airplane with her little finger and thumb extended at opposite ends, then a big recoil and a mighty "whoosh!" through the air followed by a loud giggle. I believe Lindsey loved the sensation of flying. If you put her on a swing, the smile broadened with every push. I think it was the rush of air against her face and the feeling of weightlessness. Probably she got more air into her lungs that way, and in general maybe it was just good for her.

As her frustration with communication faded, Lindsey's true personality and behavior began to bloom in her interactions with us and in her playing. Like any other little girl, Lindsey sometimes emerged from the bathroom after going for a treasure hunt in Mom's makeup case. She would have on makeup, lipstick, and at least fifteen different multicolored bows and bands in her hair. She wore a big grin each time and was always proud when she could dress up or make herself up. She loved to put on our clothes for fun. She was always keen on clothes and very particular about how she dressed. Pink and white were her favorite colors, with yellow a close second.

As Lindsey got older, with continued work through EI, she began to string several signs together to make sentences. About this time her speech actually began to develop. Of course, "Mommy" and "Daddy" were the first words to come out very clearly. During this period we would see a mixture of actual speech combined with sign language. Later on we would get both at the same time. I was very proud of her ability to use this tool. Lindsey could easily sign the whole alphabet. Donna and I could as well.

Chapter Three

After a few months, the signing dropped off more and more as Lindsey got more and more chatty. We enrolled Lindsey in a developmental preschool for special needs children. In this environment, Lindsey began her affinity for learning that never went away. I remember her bonding with a nice teacher named Sherrie who noticed potential in Lindsey and developed affection for her.

Lindsey loved to create things by drawing or working with paper. She learned to read words, and later sentences, and had many books. In school through the years she was a diligent student. She was provided with speech and occupational therapy, which improved her communication. Her fine motor skills were unusually good. Lindsey could practically thread a needle and could do other things requiring fine motor skills quite well. This was not so much a learned skill as a discovered talent that was strengthened through therapy. Lindsey was also good at playing games requiring putting different shapes through keyed slots.

Her gross motor skills, however, were much later in developing. We found out years later that a series of ear infections had left fluid in her ears, and that was what had delayed her more in her speech. We had to have tubes put into her ears. I remember the day the ear tube placement was scheduled was precisely the morning that Hurricane Fran hit us in Raleigh. We had to reschedule. The procedure went fine, and we could tell that her rate of development accelerated over the next few months.

Lindsey progressed through another very good developmental preschool called Frankie Lemmon School. During this time she had some health concerns with her heart, but her education did not suffer. Lindsey did very well in spite of everything.

Liquid potassium was proving to be very challenging to take. It was during this period and just prior to entering Penny Road Elementary that Lindsey had her last big heart surgery. During that stay a pharmacist at UNC Hospital came up with some new tasteless and dissolvable potassium chloride tablets to try. We learned that we could dissolve these into peach-flavored baby food, and Lindsey ate this well if chased with lemonade. This potion is what seemed to make a big change for Lindsey, and she had many years of remarkably good luck with this medicine.

During this time period with Lindsey's speech developing we began to see that she really had a keen imagination. I used to label this as her telling "tall tales." Once when she had been wetting the bed for a couple of days straight and felt a little embarrassed about it, Donna and I went into her room and discovered it once more. We asked her, "Lindsey, why did you wet the bed again?" Almost immediately, we got a sheepish grin and a real tall tale. Lindsey said, "Big white duck from lake flew in my window and wet my bed." We laughed so hard we could not say or do anything for several seconds. Once after she went on a field trip to NC State, Lindsey told us that she had fun because she had seen "green snakes lying on rocks." Later we learned from the teacher that this was indeed another "Lindsey tale."

At Penny Road Elementary School when she was seven years old, Lindsey became known to almost the entire student body and all of the teachers. Although in a class for special children, she was allowed many opportunities to interact and mainstream with the general student body. She roamed the halls, talking to everyone, and played on the playground equipment like any other child. I have pictures of her climbing across what we call "monkey bars" and hanging upside-down. I could not believe how well she was doing. One of the teacher's aides in Ms. McInnis's and Ms. Rogers's classes was a tall, friendly former track athlete named Mr. Freeman. Lindsey loved Mr. Freeman, and his nickname for her was "Cupcake." This was one of several nicknames that stuck around.

Lindsey learned to read some, and learned other skills including cooking in a kitchen. This would later become her favorite place. Lindsey made many friends including a nice lady working in the library named Ms. Errato. She had a son at Penny Road named Anthony who was the same age as Lindsey.

There were a few bouts with viruses and illnesses that required hospitalization, but the stays were each only a few days because she recovered quickly. Taking medicine simply became a routine. It was not always easy in the mornings, but we always got through it fine.

Lindsey spent her before- and after-school time for many years at a center called Babes and Kids. There Lindsey appointed herself as the afternoon parent-child locator. She knew all of the kids' names and had learned to recognize all of their parents. When she would see a parent get out of the car and walk to the door, she would announce to the child to get ready because his or her parent was there to pick him or her up. Lindsey loved to be around small children, especially babies.

It was at Penny Road that Lindsey first became involved with Special Olympics. Her favorite events were the 50-

meter run, the standing broad jump, and the softball throw. When Batman visited the opening ceremonies one year, I videotaped her getting him a drink of water. She competed in Special Olympics for many subsequent years, and it was always wonderful to see her smile when standing on the podium getting ribbons. When Lindsey was running, you could see her mischievous eyes dancing like crazy. That always melted my heart into soup.

You have to see what Special Olympics does for these children from their perspective. It is a chance to overcome the physical prisons of their bodies for a short period and experience what the rest of us take for granted. To compete and win means overcoming obstacles through hard work. For most of these kids, reaching the finish line is like scoring a winning touchdown or soccer goal.

It was during this period that Lindsey became the most physically active she had ever been in her life. At home I built a swing set with a sliding board, and she gave it a real workout, especially climbing on the rings and swinging.

Lindsey always loved the pool when we went to the beach. She would stay in it for several hours at a time, and it never seemed to hurt her so long as we kept her coated with sun block and a hat. I think she liked the water as a weapon against evil gravity because she would just kind of bounce or hop continuously in the water.

Swimming underwater to Lindsey was to hold her nose, then dunk her head in the water like a baptism and come back up. We had Lindsey take swim lessons once in a class for special-needs kids. She still was never able to go in over her head, but she did overcome her fear of the water and never wore a life jacket again after the swim lessons.

Chapter Three

For many years and even through her sixteenth birthday, Lindsey loved for me to go out in the yard and pitch plastic balls to her. She would make contact every few pitches and smash at least two each session out into the yard a fair distance. Lindsey also loved watching movies about baseball, the latest being *The Rookie*. She loved stories about the underdog coming back to win the big game.

As Lindsey got older, she had a ritual where she would swing, then shoot basketball, then get on her little pink Schwinn bike and ride in our driveway. Another thing she would do was if she caught me working in the flower garden, she would put on her little gloves and come out to help. Every so often, Lindsey would take a short walk out the back door and down the driveway, then back onto the front sidewalk.

My most poignant memory is of Lindsey coming outside to swing while I was mowing the backyard. I think she used to do it just to ease my mind. I believe Lindsey knew I worried about her health, and it was as if she was saying, "OK, Daddy, I'm fine and I'm going to prove it!" She could swing herself very high and as near the top as any other kid. Each time coming down from the rear height a huge smile would emerge on her face. I could see it as I rounded the corner with the lawn mower. I cannot remember any other moments in life making me as happy as those.

During the Penny Road field day one May, Lindsey was photographed doing many activities including playing miniature golf, running, and having a pillow fight with the person some outsiders thought was her twin—her brother Tyler.

Chapter 4
Looking Like Tyler's Twin

When Lindsey was a little over three years old, an addition to the family arrived in the form of a younger brother we named James Tyler Alexander. I believe it was watching the end of an exciting football game on TV that triggered my wife to go into labor. Our alma mater, the NC State Wolfpack, had just won an exciting victory in a bowl game, and that was enough to do it.

We agreed not to make James a "junior" for many reasons. For example, my own brother was a "junior," and he and my father always got their mail mixed up, so we chose to avoid this problem. We decided to call him Tyler, which was a cross between my wife's family name (Tysinger) and mine (Alexander).

Tyler was a very healthy baby, and Lindsey seemed to thrive with a baby brother. The added stimulation also helped her development. After attending many football games as a family with baby Tyler, his first words were "Git em!" No doubt this was an encouragement to a pursuing defense. Lindsey loved the roar of the crowd, the band, the cheerleading, and interacting with all of the people who sat next to us, especially the lady with the wolf slippers.

By age three, Tyler's growth and speech made him look very close in size and development to Lindsey. In fact, we have scores of pictures of the two together where they look like twins. Tyler's hair was turning from a reddish tint to a blond while Lindsey's was already a darker shade of the same color. They did almost everything together, as the many pictures will testify.

Because Lindsey was physically doing pretty well during this period, they seemed to always be playing chase games like "duck-duck-goose" or dancing in front of the TV to Disney videos. Tyler was a willing playmate who loved his sister very much. I remember us taking them to the beach and pulling them both in the red Radio Flyer wagon. A man near the pool asked me if they were twins. He said, "You sure have two cute children." With her shirt on, you could not see the scars of Lindsey's surgeries, and she behaved and sounded just like a child of Tyler's exact age.

In a way this continued for a few more years. Lindsey's growth kept her a little ahead of and then even with Tyler until she reached about age thirteen. At that time Tyler's growth spurted and he passed her. Developmentally I believe that Tyler helped pull Lindsey ahead, and she also always had a little something to teach him as well, since she was an older sister. Lindsey always kept up with what Tyler was doing, where he was going, and what he should be doing—which Donna and I found very funny. "Tyler, go to your room and do your homework!" was often heard in our home.

There is a country music song on the radio that really paints a picture of my recollection of Lindsey and Tyler during this "twins" period. It says something about a carrot top (Tyler) who can barely walk with a sippy cup of milk, and then a blue-eyed blonde (Lindsey) with shoes tied wrong who has to dress herself. Then it mentions a beautiful girl (Donna) holding both of them. I can see Lindsey there with those little pink tennis shoes on the wrong feet that she insisted on tying herself, being held by Donna in one arm and Tyler being held in Donna's other arm with his partially red hair and blue sippy cup in hand. It just paints that image in my mind, and every time I hear the song on the radio I think of that picture.

All in all this was a very happy time for us, except that my father passed pretty early in Tyler's life, when he was about eighteen months old. I remember my father coming to visit us at our old home just before he got sick with cancer. He preferred to call Lindsey by her middle name, "Michelle," and even sent her a cassette tape of the Beatles "Rubber Soul" with the song "Michelle" on it. He said it made him think of her. I was touched; I never thought my dad would ever go into a music store and buy a Beatles cassette for anyone. Dad was saddened by Lindsey's heart condition but very impressed by her intelligence. He told me that she was special—that she had "all kinds of sense," as he put it.

A few months later, I remember taking Lindsey and Tyler out to the site of our new home that was under construction and watching them both running around in the footings. Also I remember Lindsey picking out the location of her room even before it was constructed. Both of these kids thrived at our new home. We consider ourselves very lucky that we were able to provide this for our kids in spite of everything that happened.

Tyler and Lindsey fought over trivial things just like any other brother and sister. However, it was Tyler who was the most protective of Lindsey. On family trips to theme parks or malls where much walking was required, it was Tyler who took the lead to push Lindsey's wheelchair around. Aside from Donna and myself, Tyler was the only other person who would take the time to give Lindsey her potassium supplement. After Donna or I made up the concoction, it was taken one spoonful at a time and chased with lemonade after each bite, taking about twenty minutes total each time. We had to do this every morning and every night, or twice a day every day of the week.

Tyler cared very much about his sister. Lindsey always got special accommodations on seating and got the front seat of the car near the heat and air conditioning. Although Tyler could sometimes be annoyed by it, he tolerated it very well and even supported her most of the time. He loved to tease her because he enjoyed her reaction. Usually when she didn't like something he was doing, she would emit a funny sound, something like a dog or bear growling followed by his name. I think he loved to hear this and did some things just to provoke it.

Chapter 5
Lindsey Tunes, East Cary Middle, and the Drill Team

When Lindsey was about three years old we noticed that music was something that really got her going. She loved to hear just about anything with a bouncy rhythm-and-blues or Latin-type rhythm. She did this little bounce and twist that I can only compare to the gopher on the movie *Caddyshack.*

At age five Lindsey could sing along with her favorite phrases in certain songs. There were several songs on the radio that really got her fired up. I decided to make a cassette tape of some of these songs. I recorded them off old record albums and the radio and made her a cassette tape she could pop into her little player. I even found a cute picture of her, made a copy of it, and cut it out and pasted it on the jacket of the tape. The tape got a title, which was "Lindsey Tunes." Even when Lindsey was as old as fifteen, we usually were forced to put the cassette into the player in our old minivan and play "Lindsey Tunes." She never grew tired of them. I still have the tape.

As Lindsey grew older she started as a fan of Britney Spears, then the Backstreet Boys and *NSYNC just like most kids. But she also favored some of the older artists like the Beach Boys and James Taylor. I can remember her singing along with "Carolina on my Mind" and "You've Got a Friend" so many times. I can still remember her version of the song being "Gone to Carolina in my, my, my mind" with two extra "mys" always thrown in. Another of Lindsey's favorites was Jimmy Buffett, especially the song "Cheeseburger in Paradise." I can remember her singing along with it on the way to school. Lindsey in general did not like music that was too loud, so we were careful who we took her to see. Our family went to outdoor concerts sometimes, and she liked them.

After Penny Road Elementary, Lindsey was assigned to attend East Cary Middle School. Like at Penny Road, Lindsey was very active, and soon just about everyone knew her. At East Cary, Mrs. Robin Kozichek was her teacher, and Mrs. K. really challenged Lindsey with nightly homework and aggressive IEP goals. An IEP is an individualized educational plan that is prepared to help children with special needs progress developmentally. I was amazed that it was all handwritten and at how much effort she put into it.

I will admit that the homework was very tough on Lindsey—and all of us—at night because by that time she was only ready for sleep. Somehow we got through it, and Lindsey did progress quite a bit academically. Her reading improved to where she would notice things on signs and read them out loud when we were riding. Mrs. K. became attached to Lindsey just like Ms. McInnis and Ms. Rogers did at Penny Road.

There was another lady at East Cary who took a special liking to Lindsey and offered her a chance to do something I never thought possible. Betsy Marlowe[*] had gotten to know Lindsey and talked to Donna and me about her trying out for the school drill team. We talked to Lindsey, and she said that she wanted to do it. I am not sure why or how, but she and another special-needs student were added to the drill team. At first I was apprehensive because I did not know if she could handle the physical rigors of this activity. My fears went away the first time I saw them perform. Lindsey learned the moves well and did a good job.

Donna figured out how to best modify Lindsey's uniform to fit her well. We have a picture of Lindsey doing one of her drill team poses in her uniform. Virtually no one could tell that she was not a perfectly healthy and genetically perfect young lady. At that moment she truly was. Oh, if we could all sometimes just freeze a moment in time. Would that not be so wonderful?

I was driving through a very nice small town named Apex a few days ago, and I still remember seeing the actual spot where Lindsey marched by with her drill team and continued at least a mile during a Christmas parade. I remembered the grass bank her brother and I sat on to cheer her on as she went by. She survived it well. The next day she was not sick with fluid retention. I had to pinch myself at our good luck and smile at the grace of God.

---

[*] This name has been changed.

It was during this time at East Cary Middle that one of Lindsey's classmates named Brian Buckley became a very close friend. Anthony Errato from Penny Road was at East Cary Middle as well, but their friendship would develop later.

In the late spring, another very special gift from God arrived in the form of baby Matthew, Lindsey's second brother.

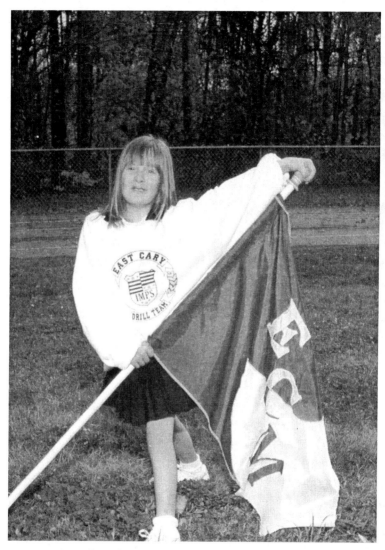

Lindsey on the drill team, 2000.

Chapter 6
Helping Raise Matthew and Going to Grandma's

If Tyler was a like a twin to Lindsey, then it could also be said that Matthew was viewed by Lindsey as her baby. Lindsey was absolutely delighted when he was born. Like when Tyler was born, there was a very good period following the birth and return home where she was not sick at all.

Matthew was born at Rex Hospital just like Tyler and Lindsey. Matthew had very thick, dark black hair at birth, which was in definite contrast to our other two children. The pregnancy and delivery went well. We picked out the name Matthew from our baby name book because it meant "gift from God." We truly felt that he was.

From the beginning, Lindsey could be seen actively participating in his care. She would assist in preparing bottles and even pick him up and sit down and feed him the bottle. Lindsey would help change his diapers. Matthew tells us now that his sister Lindsey taught him many things. He never says much, but when he does the sentiment is more powerful than ten thousand words. He simply gets a sad look with his eyes welling up and says, "I miss Lindsey." With Tyler getting older and staying more and more involved with activities outside the home, it was Lindsey who spent the most time with Matthew when Donna and I did work around the house.

Lindsey would break out the arts and crafts, paper, scissors, and games, or they would play computer games together. Matthew learned from Lindsey how to make fine paper airplanes. Once, in the hospital during a recovery period, Lindsey made about six paper airplanes and hurled them out into the hallway at nurses as they came by her room, giggling each time. I have to admit that Lindsey's paper airplanes were always flight-worthy. At home, they almost always sailed all the way from the kitchen through the dining room and into our bedroom.

Occasionally, we would see Lindsey sitting up on the couch with Matthew and reading him a book. By age thirteen Lindsey could read children's-level books very well, and her speech was fine and not an impediment at all. One notable book was *Why Benny Barks*. Listening to her read this book was like seeing all the earthly constraints of bad health and Down syndrome all drowned out by the sweet music of her voice ringing out the words on each page.

Lindsey would sometimes teach and play with Matthew for as long as three hours straight while Donna and I were busy working around the house. She had a very good work ethic. I cannot recall seeing Lindsey go into the living room or anywhere and just sit to rest for long periods of time. This girl had to be busy unless she was sick.

Lindsey's pattern on the weekend was simple. I would get her up around 7:00 A.M. for medicines, then allow her to go back to sleep. Around 9:00 A.M. sharp we would always hear a knock on the wall outside the kitchen. She loved for us to ask, "Who is it?" Then she would spring into the room yelling, "Boo!" Usually she had already changed into her clothes for the day.

Lindsey typically ate breakfast by about 9:30 A.M., and then she would go to work on arts and crafts, puzzles, or playing with Matthew. Often she and Matt would watch a video while doing something else. Then she would stop for lunch, and then would go back to work until we went out to eat for the evening. Going out to eat on Saturday evenings was an event Lindsey looked forward to all week long. This was usually a two- to three-hour excursion, so we often went as early as 3:30 P.M.

Lindsey would make as many as three separate trips through the food line at the buffet restaurant where we usually ate. She liked to eat slowly, chewing well, and taking in all that was going on around her. If the staff sang "Happy Birthday" to someone, this was highly entertaining to her. I often had to just sit with Lindsey for the last hour, drinking a cup of decaf while she finished eating a plate of salad and fruit for dessert. I used to kid her that she ought to be sitting at a sidewalk café in Paris; she would be right at home.

At night after eating, Lindsey took her medicines again and brushed her teeth. Lindsey took very good care of her teeth. When she had a loose tooth, she would wiggle it persistently until it just fell out. She pulled every single one of her baby teeth by herself; one of these came out while we were watching a movie in a theater.

After brushing, she would put on her pajamas, and then we would usually watch TV together as a family. She always fell asleep by about 8:00 P.M., and I had to put her in her bed, always saying a prayer and singing a song for her. The song was a modification from one I heard on the movie *Three Amigos* written by Randy Newman called "My Little Buttercup." I sang this to her every night for years. One day while at Target I saw the DVD and bought it. This became one of our favorite Saturday night movies to watch. Lindsey loved comedy.

On school nights the ritual was similar, except morning medicines happened at 6:30 A.M., school was the activity during the day, and supper was at home, and there was no TV at night before bedtime. Oh yes, and in the afternoons, Lindsey knocked on the wall when she got home from school around 6:00 P.M. and then sprang into the room yelling, "Boo!"

It seemed very natural and right for us to have three children. Everything seemed to fit. Matthew simply added another dynamic which helped motivate us all along. Personality-wise he is closer to Lindsey than Tyler. Matt has much of Lindsey's outgoing personality. Matt is a happy-go-lucky kid who loves to be around other people. Tyler is a happy guy who likes a tight but close circle of friends. He is less likely to explode or entertain in a crowd of people than Matthew, but every bit as wild inside the house or around his closest friends. Lindsey could be a little like both of them, but in general loved a crowd.

Chapter Six

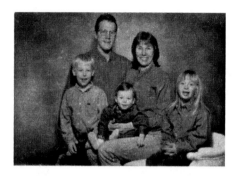

First family picture with Matthew, 1997.

Lindsey loved to travel with her brothers to Lexington, North Carolina, to stay at her grandparents' house. Her grandfather Rayvon is a very good cook who creates a lot of his own recipes. Once there, Lindsey liked to put on her apron and hang out with him in the kitchen.

Lindsey's grandmother Caroline paid her a lot of attention and kept her in top notch fashion by snatching up bargains at nearby stores. Thanksgiving and Easter were probably Lindsey's favorite times to go there. Many times Lindsey would call her grandparents a month ahead of Thanksgiving just to place her order for the holiday meal. Once when they failed to make cooked apples, she was very disappointed and expressed her disapproval: "Where's the cooked apples? Uggggh!" Her arrival ritual at their front door at Thanksgiving was to knock, followed by a greeting: "What's to eat?"

On Thanksgiving there was always turkey, dressing, sweet potato pudding, corn, and green beans, and Lindsey loved it all. On Easter she always got to color hard-boiled eggs and hunt for Easter eggs in the backyard. Lindsey

loved talking and teasing with her Uncles Charles and
Gary, Aunts Tammy and Robin, and cousins Dawn, Alison,
Drew, and baby Emily. Lindsey especially loved to boss
her Uncle Charles and earned the nickname "boss lady"
from him. Charles used to say that Lindsey ate only one
meal a day—"all day long!" Above all, Lindsey knew she
was loved by everyone there, and they miss her almost as
much as we do.

Chapter 7
Boyfriend Brian

When Lindsey started at East Cary Middle, she made an acquaintance named Brian Buckley who sat next to her every day. At first they were just classmates who saw each other daily and interacted with each other. By the time Lindsey reached the eighth grade, she and Brian had become much closer. They actually looked forward to going to school every day so they could see each other. They went to the eighth grade dance together.

About the time they started high school together, we started getting phone calls at home from Brian requesting to talk to Lindsey. These conversations were pretty hysterical, but mostly because they were just too cute. I called them "Desi and Lucy" because they would discuss things and sometimes argue when Lindsey would start telling Brian how it was to be. Brian is of Italian descent with handsome features and dark black hair, while Lindsey was fair-skinned with light-colored hair. When they were on the phone I did not eavesdrop on purpose, but occasionally they would talk loudly enough that I could not help overhearing them. To hear them talk, you would think they were two regular teenagers, not two kids with Down syndrome. Brian is also a very strong-willed kid, and they went back and forth as other couples do.

I could tell that Lindsey loved to talk to Brian because she would always smile real big right before they hung up. I believe this was very good for both of them developmentally. If Lindsey had just physically had a better heart I think those two may have been married one day.

In fact there was an occasion later in high school before Lindsey's last illness where Brian gave Lindsey a ring and they kidded that they were going to be married. Lindsey even joked that they were going to have kids, but Brian vehemently argued "No kids! No kids!" Forget about the fact that the ring wasn't a diamond—the intent and spirit behind it was as genuine as the rock of Gibraltar. I was told that sometimes while Lindsey was waiting for the school bus, Brian's parents would come to pick him up at the curb and she would actually run up to him while he was in the car and make them roll the window down so she could kiss him good-bye on the cheek. At school on Halloween Lindsey dressed up as what she described to everyone as "Batmanwoman" with the offset eyes in the mask while Brian was Elvis. They posed for pictures together.

Lindsey and Brian liked doing fun things together like playing video games. A sense of humor and being able to have fun is something any marriage counselor will tell you is a prerequisite for a long relationship together. They cared about each other for the right reasons, which is a lesson for us all. I think that they had a deeper relationship, prizing just being together above all else. When you ask nothing more than just to be around someone and that makes you happy, then you must know that is real. I believe this is what Brian and Lindsey had. Some folks call these kinds of unions being "soul mates." If that is so, well, they will be forever, no matter what.

We have pictures of Brian and Lindsey taken for the eighth grade prom when she was fourteen years old. These pictures were simply outstanding. They looked so good all dressed up together. You could see that for these moments they had truly escaped the world of being a step behind and gone right into the mainstream.

One thing I have learned is that for what these kids lack in academic intelligence, they compensate in situational intelligence. They know by one look at your face or by your spoken word what is going on and how to correctly perceive emotions. When Lindsey was in the hospital the spring before her last illness, she made me go out and buy Brian a birthday present. This unselfish consideration of others while being seriously ill really touched my heart. But then, rarely a day went by that she did not do that to me.

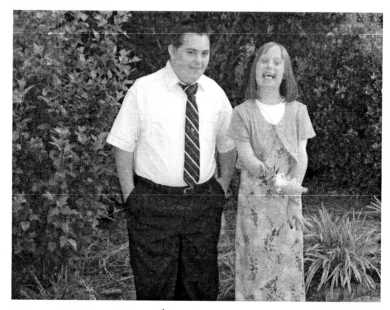

Brian and Lindsey before 8th grade prom, 2001.

Chapter 8
Prissy Pot in the Red Truck

Some of my fondest memories come from driving Lindsey from point A to point B in our red Ford Explorer, which she called the "red truck." She loved to go places. Whether it was riding to the YMCA before school or to school directly, or just to run to the store to get some gas (and SweetTarts), she was always happy to be riding. I loved to see her in my front seat and to see her smile. Lindsey even looked forward to me picking her up to go to get her blood checked. She simply accepted it. In fact, she looked beyond that and saw that it was an opportunity to go somewhere with me and to maybe get a take-out lunch she could bring back to school to eat. She relished the simple things. She overlooked what the rest of us consider significant issues.

Medicine runs were frequent. I can remember Lindsey going with me many times to the drive-thru at Eckerd

Pharmacy to pick up her medicines. In fact, most of the workers there knew her by name. I can remember on one occasion when it was about 9:30 P.M. and we picked up medicine at the drive-thru at Eckerd. Mary was working the window. Lindsey looked at her from the passenger side and hollered "Hey, why are you guys here so late? Are you homeless?" The way she said it was so funny, and it cracked Mary and me up quite a bit.

One other thing Lindsey absolutely loved was to ride with me in the truck to get take-out seafood on Sunday nights. We did it almost every Sunday for about eight years. Most of the time we went around 6 P.M. We always tuned in to 94.7 and listened to the "PineCone Bluegrass Show," which only airs at that time and day. There was something about heading up Blaney Franks Road, then Ten-Ten Road, and listening to the bluegrass music, watching the dip of the sun, and seeing that girl's face beaming joy that was intoxicating. She was happy because this was our special time.

Once at the restaurant, Lindsey often talked to a lady named Terry who worked there. I think Lindsey had the ability to make bonds with people. She expected them to be there for her. She wanted to see them just to see how they were doing and to connect. Another lesson for us—we all need to just connect. We're all so busy; we need to just stop and take time to connect before it's too late. Our time with one another is so short.

Lindsey and Donna used to kid each other frequently when we would both arrive at the house coincidentally at the same time. Lindsey would call out to Donna, "Hey, you prissy pot in the red car!" Donna was driving the red convertible and she would call back, "Hey, you prissy pot in the red truck!" Lindsey always giggled loudly when she heard this and her eyes would dance. I always thought this was funny the way Lindsey loved to pick with people in good nature. As I grew older and my hair thinned on top, Lindsey began to call me "bald-headed boy." She would say, "You are bald-headed boy," and then follow that with a loud giggle. I suppose that when I started getting my hair cut shorter that didn't help any.

Lindsey liked to go with her mom to get her hair cut, and she became friends with a lady named Kerry and formed a strong bond. Kerry talked a lot to Lindsey while she cut her hair. Lindsey hated it when her bangs got cut because sometimes the hair would go into her mouth and she'd do her classic "Uuuuugggggghhhhh" animal noise. Kerry was always very patient with her. Afterwards Lindsey knew we would probably stop at the pizza restaurant nearby, so it was something she always looked forward to.

One funny thing Lindsey did on occasion was right after you had made a strong remark or claim about something. She would come up and stand right in front of you and say "Look me in eye!" Then when you tried to look her in the eye she would cross them and then roll them up to the ceiling and all around, then start laughing. It always seemed to be funny, as her comedic timing was usually very good.

Lindsey loved Halloween and dressing up to go door to door to collect candy. Her approach was always the direct one. Instead of saying, "Trick or Treat!" she would say, "Give me some candy!" But then she always followed it with a loud "Thank you!"

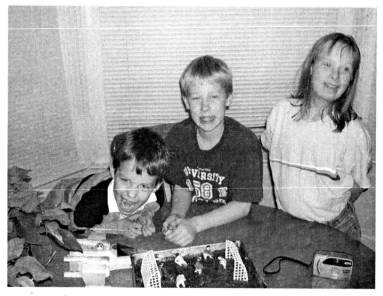

Tyler's 10th birthday with Matthew and Lindsey, 2000.

By far Lindsey's favorite trip out was to go with her mom to Food Lion and BJ's Warehouse for groceries on Sunday afternoons. To this day, there is a note preserved on the dry erase board that Lindsey wrote the day before she went in the hospital—a reminder to go both places. Lindsey knew the locations of all of the foods in both stores and which aisles to go down. Sometimes she would start and even finish writing the grocery list for her mom.

To Lindsey it was like a celebration to go into these stores and select food to eat. This was nothing to take too lightly, in her opinion. Every item caused excitement. She would always say, "Yummy!" at the sight of each food she wanted. Lindsey liked the merchandise and everything in BJ's. To her it was just a fun time. If Lindsey ever misbehaved, all we had to do was threaten to take away her trip to Food Lion and BJ's, and usually that was all it took to straighten her up.

If Lindsey had her mind set that she was going to go somewhere specific or do something in particular, then she could be impatient if there were delays. Her eyes would dance around back and forth and she would say, "You are holding up all the progress!" with a little giggle to follow.

Lindsey had some rituals that had to be followed, especially at night in the house. The sunroom door had to be closed. The ice machine on the refrigerator had to be set on "crushed ice" or she would stop in the hallway on the way to bed and reset it. Something else Lindsey liked to do was to slip secretly into our bedroom and reset Donna's alarm clock. The next morning when the alarm failed to go off or went off at an odd time, Donna would say, "All right, Miss Lindsey, quit messing with my alarm clock!"

Chapter 9
Saturday Night at the Movies

On Saturday nights, Lindsey loved to come back from eating and just crash on the couch and watch a movie with the rest of the family. Lindsey was the one who picked out the couch in the store. It had a section on one end that seemed to be designed just for her. She even lay on it and went to sleep in the store. We knew this must be the one, so we bought it. It turned out to be perfect for our living room.

On Saturday nights we usually let Lindsey decide what to watch, because in general what she chose seemed to fit the mood of the whole family for some strange reason. She had several favorite movies, and we would watch them many times over and over. Looking back, they were always good. Maybe it was because she was there to laugh with us. Perhaps it was her laughter that we enjoyed more than the movies.

The first two *Home Alone* movies were two of her very favorites. Lindsey knew many lines from both movies. She would walk around the house and quote scenes from them, which was hilarious. She would come up to me and tell me something like, "Buzz, your girlfriend, woof!" and I would crack up. She knew and sang the "Cool Cat" scene in the second movie as well. Lindsey took a strange liking to John Candy who was in *Home Alone, Rookie of the Year,* and *Uncle Buck,* which we also watched many times. He is probably entertaining her in heaven now for sure.

Luckily DVDs came out in time for Lindsey to watch them for a couple of years. Her absolute two favorite DVDs that we used to all watch were *The Rookie* and *The Three Amigos. The Rookie* was about a guy about forty years old who is a high school coach who discovers he can throw a fastball at ninety-five miles an hour. It is the part about the underdog who comes back and makes it to the big leagues that I believe attracted her. Perseverance was definitely one of her trademarks. *The Three Amigos* was just plain silly, which is why she loved it. She thought the wacky singing and acting were hilarious. I think she liked it when the Three Amigos did their "amigo salute" with the twist and cough at the end.

We always watched the TV show *Touched by an Angel* on Saturday nights. Lindsey loved watching that show, especially the song at the introduction. She used to sing "Walk with me!" along with the TV.

Probably her favorite videos to watch alone were *Toy Story,* parts 1 and 2, *Shrek,* and *Lilo and Stitch.* There were parts she had memorized that she would parrot back to us at random times. This was always entertaining and one of the things I miss so much about her.

Now when we watch a new movie for the first time, we always decide whether or not Lindsey would have liked it. It's not a very hard determination to make. Lindsey liked two things—happy family situations and comedy. If the movie or show had both, then it was really good to her. When I think about it that way I feel exactly the same way.

Chapter 10
Going to Church

Lindsey often guided us into doing new things for the better. It was her idea while in grade school for us to start recycling plastic, paper, and glass. We still do this to this day.

Lindsey is the one who got us all to eat healthier. We cut back on our salt and fat intake and ate lean meats, seafood, and more vegetables.

When she left us, we felt a little clueless because she so frequently asked what we were going to do and helped us figure it out. She planned many of the meals and helped with the grocery list. We planned many activities to accommodate her. We chose to include Lindsey far more often than to split up and exclude her. Unless it was too hot or we couldn't take a wheelchair where long walks were required, in general she went where we went.

She talked about us needing to go to church, so we did and still do. I know Lindsey did not pay attention to everything said at church, but she caught all of the big points and clung to them. Lindsey talked about Jesus and God like they were what we all needed. Lindsey would say sometimes, "Jesus is good for you and God is good for you." Sometimes she gave me cold chills with her declarations because they were so full of honest, simplistic conviction. I thought, well, here is a gift from God with a little God built in. I don't believe she was parroting anyone this time. These were notions born in her little head of her own reasoning.

Lindsey liked to dress up for church. We would drive up and I would drop her, the boys, and Donna off in front so the walk would be short. Sometimes she wanted to walk in with me, so she would not get out of the car; this frustrated Donna sometimes. We dealt with it.

I remember Lindsey wearing her little purple dress many times to church. I found it humorous and ironic one time when we sat down next to a lady who coincidentally had exactly the same dress on in an adult size. I remember thinking they looked cute together in their purple dresses.

One of my favorite stories of Lindsey was when Donna and I had taken a rare trip alone for our anniversary and Lindsey was visiting my brother and sister-in-law's church. Her Aunt Tammy had to take her out because it was time for her medicine. As the story goes, Lindsey simply walked up front to the preacher and asked for the microphone. She then grabbed the microphone and told the congregation, "Jesus loves you and God loves you. Jesus is in your heart and God is in your heart." Then she handed the microphone back to the preacher and walked out. Reportedly several people started crying, some laughed, but all of them were touched that day by a little girl with a bad physical heart and a huge spiritual heart.

Lindsey never discriminated against anyone. To her, everyone was someone to be loved so long as they showed love to her. People who were mean she simply shied away from, but she did not care about their skin color or their choice of clothes. In fact, Lindsey's choice of dress was often just to mix a bunch of colors. In a strange way it seemed to match, but was always reflective of her personality.

I have never before seen such a mix of humanity as I did at Lindsey's funeral service There were over two hundred people of every ethnic mix and background, all focused on one thing: Lindsey's life. There were people from both my family and Donna's family, almost every one of Lindsey's school teachers, her doctors, some nurses, engineers, youth counselors, special needs children, skilled soccer players, young people, old people, and many people she just came to know. It seems as though she accomplished something that many churches and politicians cannot do and money cannot buy. She brought all of these kinds of people together for a common cause. She even managed to bring many NC State Wolfpackers and UNC Tarheels together! How many people can do that in today's world?

I am forever grateful to Reverend Rick Clayton for his words at the service.

Chapter 11
Passion for Art and Puzzles

I believe Lindsey got her passion for art and puzzle working from both of her parents but even more so from Donna on the puzzles. By the time she was sixteen years old, she owned about eight different 100-piece puzzles, three 500-piece puzzles, and even a 1000-piece puzzle. She had worked them all. Lindsey's favorite way to spend a Saturday or Sunday afternoon would be to get out three or four puzzle boxes, put in a favorite movie video, then sit on the floor and work one puzzle after another. Sometimes if she was on a roll, she could work two or three 100-piece puzzles completely during one movie. I found it simply amazing that she even had the mental dexterity to do it, but to have the drive and energy to enjoy it in the process again and again was downright inspiring.

I remember reading that as adults we utilize only a small percentage of our brains in our daily activities. Lindsey must have utilized 75 percent of hers, because she was only happy to be working it constantly during the day. When she was not working puzzles, she was either drawing or creating something by crafting paper. We had a book of origami projects and paper airplanes, and she would sometimes sit down by herself with it and figure out how to make something new. Lindsey also had access to a book of origami projects at school. Two of her favorite projects were to construct a hat made of newspaper and a paper tie. She delighted in making the whole class wear both.

I remember teaching Lindsey how to construct a four-fingered paper puppet that most kids in my generation called a "cootie trap." Some kids just never get how to make these because you have to make several folds from the corners a certain way, then flip it over and do different folds and a little fold-out maneuver to get it right. Lindsey picked it right up and never forgot how to make them. She made many of these for Matthew over the last few years.

Once in middle school, Lindsey's speech teacher introduced her to playing checkers in order to teach her the concept of taking turns. Lindsey got so good at checkers that she began beating the speech teacher.

Lindsey's drawings were not sophisticated, but they all tended to reflect her outlook on life—optimism, hope, and happiness through the colors of the rainbow. Lindsey loved to match one bright color in contrast to another in bands. In my office I have a watercolor she did for Father's Day in June of the year that she passed. It says, "**FAThers day TO JiM From Lindsey.**" The first five words are different colors. Her name has almost a different color for each letter. There are seven-banded rainbows painted in each corner. There is a small heart drawn next to my name with the word "**Love**" in red written under it. When I look at this I can see the purest form of expression emanating from it. Quite simply, it makes my heart melt to look at it. I just do not have a better way of putting it.

Sometime during the month of June or July in the same year, Lindsey drew another picture that we really did not pay much attention to, but it showed up in some papers after her death. It was clearly a drawing of an angel. We have this on display in Lindsey's room.

Chapter 12
Mama's Helper

One of Lindsey's favorite places had to be the kitchen. She loved to cook spaghetti and omelets, and she had her own cookbook. Lindsey was not a bit afraid to find a new recipe and try to cook it. For the most part there was nothing in the instructions of her children's cookbook that she could not understand.

If Donna was making a dish that required some mixing, Lindsey always wanted to do it. If we were making spaghetti, she would brown the hamburger. If I had to make hamburgers, Lindsey was the one who made the patties. She had learned how to roll the hamburger into little balls, and then press them into patties between two pieces of waxed paper. She did this without exposing her skin to the hamburger, but I always insisted she wash her hands afterwards anyway.

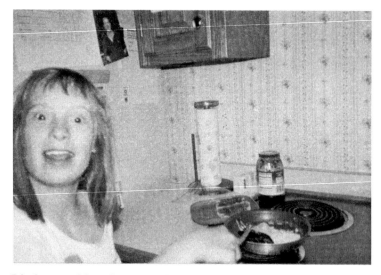

Lindsey cooking cheese omelette, 2002.

Lindsey loved to turn the oven timer off and clear it any-time it went off when Donna was cooking. Sometimes she forgot to tell her mom!

Recently we found a picture that we never knew we had of Lindsey cooking a cheese omelet and looking over her shoulder with slight surprise and excitement at the camera. Clearly she was in her element at that moment because there is a big smile on her face.

Lindsey loved cooked onions and garlic. She would have me sprinkle garlic on just about anything. Another love was pickles. We had to limit her on that because of the sodium, but I learned very recently from one of her classmates that she would go on pickle binges at school.

It was not uncommon for Lindsey to go get paper and start a grocery list for her mom on her own. She knew the drill. She would check the refrigerator, the cabinets, and the freezer, then make the list for the entire week. In general Donna only had to add a few things to complete it.

Lindsey would sometimes take initiative to empty the kitchen trashcan and put in a new liner. She was also very good at making pitchers of lemonade. Sometimes if she knew we were going to have a meal at home, she would get out dishes and set the table. After someone washed the dishes by hand, she tried to rinse them herself. But usually she would leave suds on them, so we always had to check them.

Lindsey used to help her mama clean the house. Her favorite chore was to clean the windows. Lindsey later did part time work at Golden Corral and sometimes wiped tables and cleaned windows there.

Lindsey would frequently use my cell phone to call her mom on the way home from the YMCA after school just to ask what we were going to have for supper. If there were clothes in the dryer, Donna would tell Lindsey (not me) because she was far more reliable at remembering to get them out and fold them.

Her favorite three places to shop were pretty close to each other. BJ's Warehouse, Kohl's, and Food Lion were stores where Lindsey could always see things that she would enjoy. BJ's was especially fun to her because they had clothes, toys, and food all in one place. Kohl's was a place she was familiar with because she had worked there part time folding and hanging up clothes. When I went with Donna and Lindsey to Food Lion it always amazed me how Lindsey knew where everything on the grocery list was in the store. She would say, "Over here." Lindsey not only went to the correct aisle but she would pinpoint the item and pick it up and put it in the cart. Someone else had to push the cart.

During the last year, we had to use her wheelchair in places that required a lot of walking. For whatever reason, this was never the case in Food Lion. She summoned up energy from somewhere and would zoom through the whole store. This never changed even in the very last months.

Chapter 13
High Achiever for the Queen Bee

Lindsey was blessed with good teachers throughout school, but in high school she had one who not only motivated her in the classroom but also through exposure to work. Lindsey called Tracy Serviss the "Queen Bee" because she was always in charge. It was Tracy who provided her with the opportunities to work at the Special Olympics office packing and sealing envelopes, Kohl's folding clothing, and Golden Corral washing windows and cleaning tables. She encouraged Lindsey to gain skills such as counting money and leading science experiments. Tracy took a special interest in all of her students, and it is certain that they are achieving things academically and socially under her supervision that they would not have otherwise accomplished.

Staying busy was never an issue for Lindsey. That was her natural state unless she was feeling too sick for it, which was pretty rare. At school, Lindsey became the ruler in the kitchen during cooking class—at least after they split her and another headstrong young lady into different groups. It seems that Lindsey and Leah had been actually fighting over who was going to control the big cooking spoon. This must have been like getting King Arthur's sword pulled out of the stone.

Lindsey liked to get everything situated where she wanted and would bark out orders to everyone else. Once when she got to operate a bread machine in the main school kitchen, they practically had to drag her off of it to go back to class. She even earned the job of making cookies for the student body every morning in the cafeteria. I used this as leverage on some days when we would be running a little behind. I would say, "C'mon Lindsey, you don't want to be late for making the cookies." More times than not, she would perk up a little.

About once a month she would have a day where she could not wake up enough to take all of her medicine quickly enough, and I would be nearly late for work. Tracy later told me that they could always tell how well Lindsey took her medicine by how soon she arrived for school. On one occasion, Lindsey came in to class a little late and said, "Daddy used a bad word but he still loves me." If I ever did, I pray that God will forgive me, for I would have slain any dragon for that girl.

Lindsey was also close to the teaching assistants, Ms. Sykes and Ms. Balmer. Ms. Sykes sometimes gave Lindsey rides to after-school care when the bus broke down. I could always tell that she cared very much for Lindsey, and I know that she will never forget her.

Chapter Thirteen

Lindsey became a helper to Ms. Balmer in teaching sign language to a student in the class. Lindsey had learned signing when she was very small because of her ear infections that further delayed speech development. Lindsey absolutely loved being able to help with this. Many times after lunch Lindsey would race Ms. Balmer in a speed walk back to class just to be the one to get the sign language book out.

Perhaps because of her electrolyte medicine and her layers of clothing, Lindsey seemed to always carry a high amount of static electricity. For some reason, Ms. Balmer always seemed to be the recipient of the static discharge. Therefore, Ms. Balmer's nickname for Lindsey became "Shocky."

At home it was not uncommon for Lindsey to show off some of her signing and talk about what she had done that day. She was always proud when she could do something to help someone else. Two funny things Lindsey did with sign language that she could never correct were that she always did the sign for "telephone" upside-down, and the sign for "house" always had a round motion. Some of the students thought she was saying "round house."

Lindsey sometimes entertained the class with her imitation of an elephant. She would let one arm hang down in front and then put her mouth on the other arm to make a muted sound that imitated an elephant. I suppose I have to claim some responsibility for that. OK, I admit it—and the pig sound, too.

During this period Lindsey continued to participate in Special Olympics, and I marveled at how good she was at bowling. She had better form than I did! I am pretty sure she bowled in the eighties without using rails. Lindsey took home three blue ribbons during her last spring competition.

Under different heart circumstances, with her drive and competitive nature, she would have certainly played soccer or other more vigorous sports. I miss our foosball games where she would give me a run for the money, but I must admit that I usually let her win. On occasion she would burn me when I was really trying, though.

Lindsey was very competitive. Even during the times when she used her wheelchair at school after a hospital recovery, her PE teacher tells me that she would suddenly just bolt from the wheelchair and start participating in the PE class with the rest of the kids.

Lindsey still holds the record for the most money collected for a local charity in about two hours. She had gone with some class members to collect for an organization called Knights of Columbus. It seems that while Tracy was providing instruction on the proper way to approach potential contributors, Lindsey had already run up to several and said, "Give me some money!" Apparently her direct approach worked because she collected $147 during that time.

When I look at Lindsey's school notebook, I realize that she was starting to accelerate a bit in her learning towards the end, even though her heart was worsening. She was able to correctly transpose logical statements and handle money, and her reading and speech were getting better and better. At home Lindsey would surprise us by using some bigger words that we had not heard her say before like "desperate" and "ridiculous." Her vocabulary was definitely expanding. I was always amazed at how she could sit down at the computer, boot it up, use different software, and then shut it down seamlessly. She liked to use Print-Master® software to create her own greeting cards and even mailed some out to her friends Brian and Kelly. She would also pull up a program called Deer Hunter, and she became a master at bagging eight-point bucks on the computer.

Lindsey even commented that she wanted to attend college with her cousin Dawn. I remember wondering if they had a cooking class at Wake Tech she could attend. She once did pretty well in a mainstream photography class at East Cary Middle. I think her teachers and classmates read into this that physically she was also doing pretty well. In fact the opposite was true. Deep down I suspected it, but chose to believe like everyone else that the little girl who could would just keep on going. And for such a long time, she did.

I saw Lindsey's determination and drive as being similar to my mother Julia, who died in her mid-fifties, also at an early age. Mom fought cancer for five years, taking chemo and still working to keep us all going. She always reached out to help others and kept her sense of humor. When I think of her, I think of "strong-willed and loving"—very near to what her granddaughter was. Mom always talked of wanting grandchildren. Free from pain and sickness, they now have each other forever.

Chapter 14
Planes, Cruises, and Buzz

When Lindsey was fourteen and fifteen years old, we had an opportunity to do some things that I will forever cherish. As humans we tend to look back and think how we wished we had done something different. I am no exception, and I beat myself up pretty bad about events in the hospital at the end. Finally I realized that God's plan was done and there were signs indicating that this was inevitable in those last months. The little cough that Lindsey had the last two years was actually a sign of congestive heart failure. Lindsey did have days where she appeared sluggish and tired, but she was very strong-willed and did not give in to it very much.

Truth is, you miss people who leave you. You search, dream, and even scheme of ways to fool yourself into wishing them back. Well, I think Lindsey's Uncle Charles summed it up for me nicely. He says, "I know beyond a doubt that I will be seeing that girl again someday."

Some things I look back on with no regrets and no wish to have done anything differently, especially our family trips with Lindsey. When Lindsey was fourteen, we went on a Disney cruise and Lindsey took her first plane trip. She sat right next to me and was not scared in the least. I was a little apprehensive because I did not know how her body might react to the altitude or possible turbulence planes sometimes experience. But the trip went fine. In fact, Lindsey was fascinated at the Orlando airport with the moving sidewalks. To her this was great. She walked up and down them about ten times.

Our cruise was so much fun because of her. We usually took the wheelchair with us when we went on outings, since she could not walk long distances because of her heart. But after we got situated on the boat and Lindsey got her bearings, we never got the wheelchair out again. I had requested and gotten a suite near the pool. She had no problem going from the suite to the pool, restaurant, or theater.

Lindsey had pictures taken with the Disney characters, and I made camcorder video of her having fun, dancing and continuing to interact with the characters. We also got a small refrigerator for her medicines, so storage and access were no problem. I worried some about the pitching of the boat, but it wasn't so bad and it did not bother her much. She was excited and glad to be there and we were so happy to have her there with us. Matt and Tyler had such a blast. We have pictures of Lindsey, Matt, Tyler, and me playing Ping-Pong on the deck of the boat. Lindsey most liked the good food, shows, and the party at each place we visited at mealtime.

In the spring we went to Busch Gardens in Williamsburg, Virginia. That was also a very fun trip. Lindsey had to ride in the wheelchair, but enjoyed the beautiful scenery and even some rides. We toured historic Jamestown, and Lindsey loved seeing the restored Indian village and the cooking demonstrations.

In the early summer of that year we visited Tweetsie Railroad in Boone, North Carolina. We got some great pictures of all three kids in an old frontier wagon, and Lindsey loved the train ride around the mountain. She also liked the singing and dancing at the shows. We were blessed by the absolutely gorgeous weather that day. I rode the chairlift down the mountain with Lindsey at my side. Life was sweet.

Our beach trip to Emerald Isle in North Carolina in the midsummer was great. We had the grandparents, Aunt Tammy, and Uncle Charles there. Lindsey loved the pool at Ocean Reef. But the thing she liked the most was just drawing and doing homework inside while we were on the beach in the mornings after breakfast. This would seem weird to most people, but it was normal to Lindsey. She loved to be doing work and keeping busy. In the afternoon she would visit the pool for several hours. She always preferred the pool over the beach because she really did not like sand that much.

Lindsey would come out to the beach late in the evening for just a while and sometimes watch us fishing. I remember Lindsey holding my surf rod for a bit and catching a stingray. She was so excited! Her eyes got big and she cried, "Daddy! Daddy! Daddy! I got a fish!" We took a picture of her on the beach looking back over her shoulder. We look at it a lot today. In fact, the newspaper used that picture in an article about her. I always thought she looked healthy at the beach. Maybe it was the high oxygen content in the air or the lack of pollution. Maybe she was just real happy.

Later in the fall, when Lindsey was fifteen, we went to Disney World. We stayed at Port Orleans. This was such a great trip because we got to do everything we wanted to do. We got up and did medicines, put Lindsey in the wheelchair, and then hit the nearby food court. Tyler always pushed Lindsey in the wheelchair. Breakfast was fun because we did not have any trouble finding low-salt things for Lindsey to eat there.

Then we would take off to one of the theme parks. Luckily for us, the weather was great—not too hot or cold—so it was not stressful to Lindsey to be out for most of the day. One night I will never forget was when Donna had taken Tyler somewhere and I took Lindsey to the food court to eat. We sat at the window right next to the mill pond. The moon was full and the reflection off the water looked like something right out of a Brer Rabbit tale. She was happy and smiling while eating a salad.

The time at Magic Kingdom was truly magic. Lindsey and Matt got many pictures taken with characters and saw most of the attractions there. Lindsey's favorite was the Buzz Lightyear ride. Our whole family rode this ride three times straight. Lindsey loved trying to shoot the aliens that pop up during the ride. The more you hit, the higher your score. I have never seen her have so much fun. I thought in

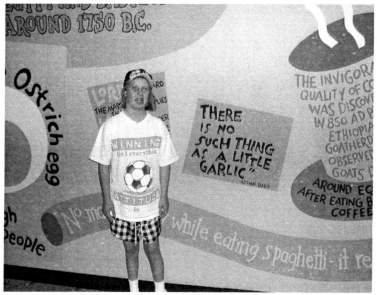

Lindsey at Disney's Epcot, 2002.

the back of my mind that this was really kind of like a "Make A Wish" trip—that it might be her last. But I figured it was just me worrying too much.

Lindsey made it through Cinderella's castle and saw a cool parade in Frontierland while she enjoyed a meal outside. She also rode the boat to Tom Sawyer's island and roamed around the fort with Matt and Tyler without the wheelchair. I do not think Lindsey much considered that she had a heart problem at that time. She was a kid sister at Disney World having a ball with her brothers. Later that evening, Lindsey got to see Tinkerbell fly from the top of the castle. For someone who had watched the *Peter Pan*

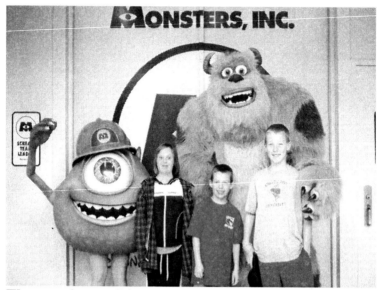

Three amigos at Disney MGM, 2002.

and *Cinderella* videos probably twenty-five times each, this was very cool.

At night we coincidentally met some friends from Raleigh at the Rainforest Café in Downtown Disney. The colors, music, and food were things Lindsey could really relate to. I remember taking some special straws with Mickey Mouse home with us from there, and then seeing Lindsey using them every so often afterwards.

The next few days we visited MGM, Animal Kingdom, Epcot, and Typhoon Lagoon. At MGM, Lindsey and her brothers got pictures made with the guys from *Monsters Inc.* Our whole family did the movie scene attraction with the fire and the flood. I remember her being just a little scared at first.

Chapter Fourteen

At Animal Kingdom, Lindsey actually got on an aerial ride at the dinosaur park and rode it twice by herself. I have video of her going by with the biggest smile, the kind that melted my heart. We also took her on the safari ride in the rover. That was a perfect mix of fun and excitement, but not too scary for her at all. A giraffe almost stuck his head in the rover, and Lindsey made one of her animal sounds at it: "Ugggghhh."

Lindsey loved animals, and I believe she plugged all of this into her memory. Lindsey also invented another sound that she made any time she saw a shirt or clothing with zebra stripes. She would go, "Zeeee-bra" while growling at the same time. It always made us laugh when she did this. I guess you had to have been there to get it.

At Epcot, Lindsey's favorite thing was the Earth exhibit with the ride through "The Land" showing innovative ways to grow food. She loved the "Food" show with the singing and dancing, and we got the coolest picture ever of Lindsey standing in front of a giant quote where someone says, "You can never have too much garlic." That was perfect for Lindsey because she loved garlic on just about everything. That one is framed in our living room.

Last, at Typhoon Lagoon, Lindsey floated down the lazy river with Donna for over one mile. After that, Donna, the boys, and I begged and finally convinced Lindsey to go down the family raft water slide. This was very scary to her at first, and she squealed a little. As we went down and she realized it was safe, she then got used to it and thought it was great fun. She did just fine. I always had to weigh whether something was going to be too exciting for her heart, but I figured if it wasn't too bad then her basic nature was that she would love it. This time I happened to be correct.

Lindsey looked a little tired on the last day, but not too bad. We went to Lego Island in Downtown Disney. She was totally impressed by the fifty-foot Loch Ness monster made of Legos in the water, and all of the other things as well. She really held up well. We had no problems with her flying back to Raleigh. She got another little burst of energy in the airport and went up and down the moving sidewalks about six or eight times while we waited for our flight home.

Chapter 15
Riding in the Boat

After Lindsey had her illness in the spring at age fifteen, I began thinking about not putting things off. We had been saving our money for over a year to buy a boat. We didn't want a big boat, but just a boat that our whole family could enjoy on the lake four miles away. Tyler and I went to the boat show and we found the one we wanted. The colors of the Stingray reminded me so much of Lindsey with the bright yellow stripes that I knew it would be named "Miss Lindsey" someday. I could see her sitting in the passenger seat messing with the radio. When I saw the word "Stingray," I thought about the one Lindsey had caught at the beach the previous summer. I remember bringing the boat home while Tyler was at YMCA camp. I took pictures of Lindsey and Matt sitting in it.

Our first time out in the boat we got Lindsey to ride in the two-person tube with Donna. She was a little scared but wanted to do it badly enough, so she got in. I remember starting off slowly and taking more time to get the boat to plane out. As I glanced back I saw that big smile break out like the sun from behind a cloud. Miss Lindsey was enjoying her ride on the lake.

When Lindsey was with us, we made sure to go no faster than fifteen or twenty miles an hour, and we were careful to avoid hitting any big wakes head-on that would scare her. We knew she wanted to be with us, and we wanted her to be there, too. The fun is not all about the speed and seeing how fast you can go against every other boat on the lake. The fun is not about how good your boat looks. The fun is about who is in the boat with you. When Lindsey was in the boat, we all wore our Lindsey glasses. Sometimes sitting on the water with the motor off in a cove with the anchor dropped and everyone eating lunch was the most fun of all.

Luckily we got to take Lindsey out about four times before her last hospitalization. The last time was just two days prior. Lindsey had asked to go out that day, and we took her and we all had a great time. Lindsey had been feeling fine, and we did not hesitate to take her out. She always rode in her "spot," which was the seat at the radio. I always had to help Lindsey step out of the boat, and she was pretty scared of the dock until she got to the middle. After Lindsey got off the boat, she was smiling as she went to the van with Donna. I pulled the boat home with the red truck. I was kicking around in my head possibly letting Lindsey drive the red truck in the backyard for about ten or fifteen feet with me right next to her. I never got around to that.

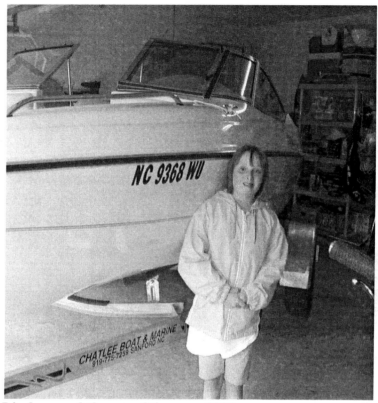

Lindsey and the new Stingray, 2003.

To be honest, things seemed to be going pretty well, and we did not expect what hit us on Labor Day that Monday when I drove Miss Lindsey in the red truck one last time to the hospital emergency room. During the ride, Lindsey told me a couple of times, "I'm going to be OK, Daddy." Then she followed it immediately by, "Do you think I'm going to be OK?" I was worried, but I told her, "You'll be fine, Lindsey."

Today one of the pictures from the day that we first brought the boat home is laminated and tied to the glove compartment above the radio. The letters on the back of our boat say "Miss Lindsey," and we really do miss her every day. I guess if I had known what was going to happen, I would have tried to protect her by keeping her inside and making sure she was very well-rested and monitored. But that is not how Lindsey wanted to live. She chose to be active and to live a quality life, placing value on every minute. That is exactly what she did and why we allowed her to pace herself in most situations.

Chapter 16
Coming Back One Last Time

I have no intention of turning this recollection of Miss Lindsey into a documentary of her last month in the hospital. Who would read it, anyway? But by the grace of God, the will of Lindsey, and a hard-working staff at UNC Hospital, we got her back one last time. It was near the end of September, and Lindsey surprised everyone by coming off the ventilator after three weeks and steadily improving for about four days. On the fourth day she could sit up, and her vocal cords improved enough for her to talk. The slight addiction to the painkillers went away, so we had her smile and her personality back. We remember her playing hide-and-seek with the pulse ox sensor, which is a small device about the size of a pea that is supposed to stay attached to a finger or toe to detect the patient's blood oxygen level. She would laugh when we found it lying underneath her and dart her eyes mischievously.

I knew she was getting better. We had her out of bed and sitting in a rocking chair, and even standing sometimes. I got to hug her, and I felt very happy. She smiled and waved at everyone in the hallway. Lindsey wanted to know how the baby in the next room was doing. She got to see both of her brothers, and she asked them how school was going. She watched *Cinderella* on the VCR. Donna and I began talking about getting a home blood pressure monitor and making plans for home.

On Sunday, September 28, 2003, Lindsey asked us, "Where's my breakfast?" that morning at 8:00 A.M. Almost immediately after that, her blood pressure dropped. That night after six hours when Donna and I stayed by her side, she left us to be with Jesus. Lindsey hated the ventilator, and there was no indication it would have made a difference had she been reconnected.

Today we realize something that it took us many months to come to grips with, and that is that she had a bad heart no one could cure and that it was God who was in control the whole time—not us, not UNC, not the nurses. The sadness on birthdays, holidays, and anniversaries poignantly stirs the pain of her being gone, but nothing takes away the happy times. We have two big picture frames full of happy pictures taken from early on through recent times. One is in our kitchen (Lindsey's favorite place) and one is in her bedroom. They keep us connected to her. Losing a child is positively the worst human experience that we've had.

For me it has brought me closer to God, but I cannot say positively that I am better off because I still do not have her. When I visit Lindsey's classmates and teachers, I cannot say they are better off, either; they still grieve after a whole year. I guess somehow getting better or stronger wasn't the point. Maybe it was simply to change our viewpoint. I do not know and will never know, at least not while I'm docked to this pier. But I do value and appreciate more what I still have, and that is a wonderful wife, two fantastic boys, and some pretty super friends, many of them Lindsey's associates.

We wonder if Lindsey isn't our guardian angel now. Like everyone else, I do not understand why so many times the good die young. I told a friend recently who lost his sister at a young age that perhaps it is so they can help the rest of us who are less good from a better vantage point, to pull us upward toward heaven.

Peace came to me one night in a dream that I cling to every day. I had been particularly upset by the coming of Lindsey's birthday. The next morning, right before I woke up, I dreamed I was in a fairly nice restaurant with a slightly dark decor and a long, open area. I was sitting at a table for four by myself, and Lindsey came be-bopping up and sat right in the seat to my left. She was smiling so big and looked so healthy and happy. She said, "Hey, Daddy!" I seized the moment. I said, "Lindsey, stand up and give me a hug!" She did, and it was so real. I told her, "Lindsey, you're so slim." Then she giggled. Immediately I woke up.

Four weeks later on a trip to Chicago, I am positive that the restaurant at my hotel looked just like the one in my dream. This was like an answer to my prayers that somehow I would be able to see Lindsey again in a dream. I feel peaceful because I know she is healthy and happy in heaven and nothing can ever harm her again. God's tender mercies sometimes come when we most need them.

Chapter 17
Newspaper Article

I am not sure why or how it happened, but a reporter with the local newspaper found out about Lindsey's passing through interactions with Athens Drive High School. It seems that they heard about Lindsey's class requesting to paint the big rock on the school grounds as a memorial. Donna and I were contacted about having an interview to contribute to a newspaper article. The article was to document some of Lindsey's life and achievements, but also to show her influence on her boyfriend and classmate Brian, and her teacher, family, and friends. The article was printed about three weeks later. Today a copy is laminated and displayed in our TV room.

To some readers, the article may have been tear-evoking and sympathetic mush. Donna and I felt like the article showed how Lindsey overcame obstacles to become a leader at home and school. Like the rock, she was strong and able to withstand the heavy weather. She had a big spiritual heart, represented by the big heart drawn on one side of the rock. But her physical heart was very weak. I think of Lindsey and hear the sound of her voice in my mind every day.

Following is the text of the article in its entirety, reprinted here with permission. I will point out one factual inaccuracy in the article and that is that Lindsey never rode in an ambulance on her last trip to the hospital. I rode with Miss Lindsey in the red truck. How could I ever forget that?

October 12, 2003
Molly Hennessy-Fiske
Staff Writer

Losing Lindsey

RALEIGH--Students who see the class gathered in front of Athens Drive High School have cause to wonder. Who gave them permission to paint the school rock? Seniors paint it for their birthdays, for homecoming and for other schoolwide events. These kids are painting it for a girl in their class. Who's Lindsey?

Some look like underclassmen, crowded around their teacher as she releases the first stream of lavender paint. One is in a wheelchair.

"Back and forth—remember how we spray the pans with cooking oil? Get close," the teacher says.

They came to the rock this Monday to honor Lindsey Michelle Alexander. Lindsey had Down syndrome, one of many disabilities shared by her classmates. She died a week before.

Classmates settled on the rock as a way to remember her. Could they paint it? They had to ask a senior adviser. Parents couldn't believe it when he said yes.

"She's not the star football player, the head cheerleader that they would do this for," Donna Alexander says of her daughter.

Fellow students and the outside world often saw the disability first. Here was a kid who didn't belong.

But to those who loved her, Lindsey Alexander was an inspiration, a bossy blonde who by age 16 had made it to school, work and Special Olympics despite lifelong heart trouble. She belonged at the heart of their past and future—walking down the aisle at church, graduations, maybe even a wedding of her own. As the outside world moves on after her death, those closest to Lindsey are still trying to imagine life without her.

The Alexanders are sitting in their suburban living room on a sunny afternoon, on the brown leather couch Lindsey picked out. They are talking about the photo collages they made for her funeral. Going through the boxes of snapshots reminded them of long ago, they say, before doctors came to tell them about Lindsey.

"That's when our world pretty much turned upside down, remember?" Jim says, rising to get the door as another flower arrangement arrives. Yep, yep, says Donna as he continues. "We went from Ozzie and Harriet to something terrible and ominous."

Lindsey was born Aug. 2, 1987, at Rex Hospital, an outwardly healthy baby after a routine pregnancy. Her parents had already seen her and held her when a doctor arrived with news. Not only did she have Down syndrome, but also a hole in her heart. The doctors could not see how she would survive infancy.

Always together

The Alexanders were just a couple of introverted engineering students at N.C. State University when they met, Donna from Lexington, Jim from Lenoir. But they took the news about Lindsey like the managers they are, at work and at home. Jim Alexander was preoccupied for about a day, then he decided not to let fears for Lindsey spoil her future. She belonged to them, and she was perfect.

As she grew and started walking and talking, first in sign language and then aloud, they learned what kind of family they would be: skintight. Lindsey was so sick—six heart operations before her ninth birthday—she pulled them closer. They made exceptions for her early on, always let her ride shotgun so she could be close to the heat or air conditioning.

"We all had to stay together," Donna says, "We got haircuts; we all had to get haircuts. We went to the dentist; we all go."

They took her and, eventually, brothers Tyler, 12, and Matthew, 7, to the beach, Busch Gardens and Disney World, where she persuaded them to board the Toy Story ride three times. Weekdays, she would make her own breakfast before Dad ferried her to school.

What did you do today, Dad, she would ask during the drive home from a YMCA after-school program. What did you have for lunch? She made him plan for the future, too. What are we doing this week, this summer? On Sundays, her father was supposed to order seafood takeout so they could go get it together and tune in to the PineCone bluegrass show on the car radio. When she got older, she was supposed to live at home so he could drive her to work.

The Alexanders went back to work two days after the funeral Oct. 1, Jim at Powerware Corp., Donna at Elster Electricity.

"How am I going to handle this new routine which doesn't include Lindsey?" Jim says. "We all looked after her... In the process I think we all needed her to be there."

The Alexanders wonder what to change and what to preserve. Where are you, Lindsey girl? Are you working on the half-solved puzzle left in the sunroom that day you woke, pale and cold, and we loaded you into the ambulance? Do you remember the month you spent at UNC Hospital's intensive care, how we held you before you died, called you beautiful and precious?

They have not moved the puzzle. Jim just can't. Donna can't get used to riding shotgun. I didn't realize how much she led us, she says. I feel her in every room, Jim says.

Last weekend, the Alexanders planted a tree in their yard, a Japanese cedar. They will see it when they leave for soccer games, for the church Lindsey loved, for the vacations and graduations she will miss. Jim already ordered a plaque they plan to strap around the trunk. "This is Lindsey's tree of life," it will say. And unlike her little bed, her tennis shoes, clothes, her very 16-year-old image, the plaque has a spring in it so it can expand, along with the space between the old life and the new.

Dreams of the future

That's Brian Buckley, dancing in the darkened stands during the Athens Drive homecoming football game. He is executing shimmies and air-punches he memorized from 'N Sync and Backstreet Boys videos, defying his sturdy frame. He's running on peanuts and adrenaline, watching his team, the Jaguars, win for the first time this year.

He's wearing their colors, nubby orange sweater and blue dress pants, both baggy. He is chilly—it's cold enough that the 16-year-old can see his breath—but he wanted to look cool. That's how he feels, and plenty of people notice.

As the marching band cranks out "Build Me Up, Buttercup," Brian can hear his three teachers cheer him on. Then one of the coolest kids to emerge from Athens Drive, professional baseball player Josh Hamilton, sits down right next to him. Hamilton starts dancing, too.

Brian can't believe it.

He doesn't notice the girl with the cell phone who stops, midconversation, to stare. Doesn't seem to see the boys laughing or the girls too busy with hair ribbons, homecoming court and sequined band sashes to say hello. Why would they? He's not in their class, not on their team or in their club.

He is not like them—he cannot read, tell the 9 from the 7 on his watch, drive a car or play football.

But like them, he wants to belong. And for a time he managed to find a girl who understood that, a girl he could belong to.

Brian and Lindsey. Their parents even had the same first names.

Yeah, he fell in love all right, but then he went and screwed it up the way any other guy would. He made the mistake of breaking up with Lindsey so he could date a new girl in class. He realized his mistake pretty quickly. He was the one who got them back together. He bought Lindsey a jewelry box with her birthstone on it, a locket with her initials and, last year, a diamond ring.

Well, it looked like a diamond to him. And it carried the same meaning.

"Deep down he thought he was going to church someday to marry her," Donna Buckley said as Brian prepared to leave for homecoming.

Nicole, a striking 19-year-old, the oldest of Brian's three sisters, nodded in agreement with her mother from her seat across the living room. She and her boyfriend used to take Brian and Lindsey on double dates. Until she graduated from Athens Drive last spring she checked up on them daily. At home, she listened to Brian talk about his budding romance and future married life.

Hearing the news

The day before the homecoming game, Brian stayed home from school. He just felt homesick, he says.

Nicole knows better.

The night before, after Lindsey's funeral, she came home from cosmetology class to find him sitting in the driveway. It was late, stars the only streetlights on Jessie Drive.

What are you doing, she asked.

Looking up at the sky, where my girl is, he said, and burst out crying. "She was my life."

His teacher had been the one to break the news to him. She took him into the kitchen attached to their classroom. Remember how Lindsey was in the hospital in February?

Yes, he did. Then she got better and they went to the Valentine's Day dance. Well, this time, the teacher said, she didn't make it.

He didn't understand. Then he did, and he started to cry.

He gathered Lindsey's pictures in his bedroom the next day and put one under his pillow. At the funeral he saw Lindsey in the casket, in the purple dress she wore to last year's prom. His locket hung around her neck.

Afterward, he turned all her pictures face down, saying, "I don't have no girl no more."

He has plenty to be frustrated about: Not being able to drive, even though he's 16; encountering boys in the cafeteria who act nice until he asks to join the hacky sack game or borrow some money; not having a girlfriend. What is he supposed to do with all this time, time he once spent playing video games with Lindsey, talking on the phone, going to dances, telling her he loved her and seeing her smile. He's exercising a little, trying to stay healthy, "because Lindsey said to."

He is painting the rock now, concentrating. He has not missed with the lavender spray paint yet. He begins to write "We love you Lindsey" with a heart shape for "love." His mother looks for the teacher and shouts:

"You might have to help him make the heart."

But it turns out Brian Buckley doesn't need any help. He can make it on his own.

Teaching the kids

Tracy Serviss is trying to referee a one-on-one basketball game in her stocking feet. Behind Brian and classmate Jakub Mitas, 17, she scoots back and forth across the slick wood floor of the Athens Drive gym, white-blond ponytail bouncing off the back of her Michigan State sweater. Brian has brought the class CD player, now blasting a Will Smith single.

"Can't nobody make it bounce like me," Smith croons.

Brian grabs the ball, runs with a swagger and shoots. It almost goes in. Brian frowns.

"I'd really like to find him a big brother," Tracy Serviss says. "I mean, he's in this house full of girls."

Her approach is all-encompassing in teaching the 10 "trainable mentally disabled" students ages 15 to 21 in the class that Lindsey attended. She gets them jobs, knows where they like to eat, when their siblings marry, or loved ones die. The queen bee, Lindsey called her.

Her students read and speak to varying degrees. Some are headstrong. They like to pretend they're dancing when they're supposed to be stacking plasticware in the cafeteria or spelling "tomato."

Lindsey could be like that. Or they try to blend in the hallway between classes and act as if they don't have a disability at all. Lindsey could be like that, too. If Serviss had her way, her kids would blend or, at least, be better received by their peers.

Does the school miss Lindsey? How many students realized a memorial broadcast on their closed circuit televisions gave the wrong last name? A few caught it before they fixed it the next day—Lindsey Wagner, it said. Like the actress Lindsay Wagner on that old television show "The Bionic Woman." Tracy Serviss laughed when she heard that. Lindsey—the bionic woman!

Brian's mom is conspiring to nominate Tracy Serviss, 36, for teacher of the year. Still, she fears the teacher spends so much time teaching that she has given up on having kids of her own. Her students are her kids, Donna Buckley says.

For Serviss, the average day goes something like this: get up, walk most of her six dogs, maybe take some of the kids out for breakfast, otherwise get to school by 7 A.M. After school, she assists people with disabilities through a state program. Unless there's a restaurant the kids want to try, a football game, dance or Special Olympics practice.

Serviss has heard her two assistants tell her she needs time for herself. They both happen to be married. She was stylish on the day they painted the rock, wearing black slacks and heels, but the only wedding she's planning is her sister's at the end of the month.

"The dances, the parties, it's fun. Plus, I don't have a boyfriend right now," she reasons. When she does, she hopes he will want to spend time with the students, too.

They belong together. She remembers how it started – growing up in New York, where she worked at summer camps for kids with disabilities. She tried to major in zoology at Michigan State, but her heart pulled her back, first to students with autism, then to those in the middle range of disability with IQs half or a third of the average student. They are so expressive, she says, yet they live without the complications of other kids their age, those she sees lingering in the school hallways using bad language.

She has taught for 15 years, five of them at Athens Drive, three of those with Lindsey. Lindsey is the second student she has lost. The other died after suffering a heart attack at home in October of Serviss' first year.

Crying and moving on

The day Jim Alexander called to say Lindsey died, Tracy Serviss could not even teach. She took her students into the classroom kitchen instead, and they spent the day cooking—learning measurements, she says. When she or her assistants started to cry, the kids would comfort them.

During the next few days she explained it to her students—what Lindsey's death means. Some people believe in heaven, she said, conscious that there are students of all faiths in her class. Lindsey's family is going to visit her grave, she told them, because that's where her body is. But her spirit is somewhere else.

I'm sad, Brian said.

"There's still going to be days when you're sad," the teacher said. "And her family will be, too."

She cried again at the funeral, and then she had to move on. She did not cry in class the day they painted the rock, when students traded silly Lindsey stories and the Alexanders showed up to claim their daughter's school picture, taken weeks before.

After they finished painting, she watched her students head for home, for the bus Lindsey would have taken to the YMCA. Then Tracy Serviss returned to her classroom, satisfied. It went better than she had expected. Brian held up, even mugged for the cameras. And the Alexanders seem to be doing well.

She began to gather her things. It was only Monday. She had work to do.

Reprinted with permission of The News & Observer *of Raleigh, North Carolina. Reproduction does not imply endorsement.*

Chapter 18
Poems Written for Lindsey

At the time of this writing it is exactly one year and two days since Lindsey's passing. Two days ago her teacher Tracy Serviss, the "Queen Bee," paid us a visit. The class had baked us cookies. They left flowers at her gravesite.

In addition, each person wrote a personal note and card telling us what they missed most about Lindsey. We also found some handwritten cards at the grave from kids at the YMCA. It made me realize that the grief over her loss does not only endure with her family members. She also endures in the minds and hearts of many others.

Following are some of the poems we have collected about her. The best poem came from a person we did not know, who had been impressed with the newspaper article. He or she sent it to the reporter, who asked if it was OK to give to us. We were very impressed with how the author used dancing to symbolize this experience so accurately. Unfortunately, I was never successful at contacting this person to obtain permission to reprint the poem. It was absolutely eloquent in its description of how Lindsey taught us not to despair in the challenges we faced but to waltz through life full of joy. I especially like the part about her life being an angel's dance and at the end her joining back with the angels. Only God makes connections like these where someone who read a newspaper article about complete strangers develops such empathy to write a work that summarizes, consoles, and inspires all at the same time. I regret that I cannot share it with everyone.

The following is a poem from a person near Lindsey's age who was in three different schools with her and also served as her YMCA counselor. Lindsey was close to Anthony and also his brother Nick, who was the director at the YMCA. Nick also cared a lot about Lindsey.

Ode to Lindsey by C. Anthony Errato II
10-1-2003

Things like these are always hard to
Try and comprehend.
It seems the world is never right
When things abruptly end.

But when I think of her right now,
Smiling up in heaven.
I picture her making animal sounds
And eating twenty-four seven.

Chapter Eighteen

I picture a heaven of marvelous things
Like her at Disneyland,
Walking and listening to Jimmy Buffet
While holding Tigger's hand.

It can make me smile to look up there,
At least when I think
That every single clothing store
Contains just white and pink.

I think of a world without diseases
But Golden Corrals are much
And also lots of arts and crafts
And applesauce and such.

It's hard to get her out of my mind
I think of her every hour
And how every day, she seemed to say
"Go home and take a shower!"

Riding with Miss Lindsey

This poem was written by one of my wife's closest friends, as written by Lindsey from beyond to her.

One More Thing by Nancy Ely-Morse
10-5-2003

Nine months you carried me in your womb
You had dreams of who I would be
God picked you because He knew
You were the perfect mother for me.

I know at first you were a little shocked
You should have seen your face
But I just giggled because I knew
You were going to learn of God's grace.

I may have done things a little slower
But you never let it show
You encouraged me and held me up
You were so proud; you had a glow.

You, and Dad, Tyler, and Matthew
My earthly family was the best
I asked God to let me stay
He insisted I needed to rest.

Please don't cry...I'm up here smiling
The food is even better than there
Someday we will be together again
At my table I've saved some chairs.

Chapter Eighteen

But there's one thing I forgot to say
I couldn't leave it undone
Thank you for the best life ever
I've had a lot of fun!

Lindsey

This poem I wrote myself because I was grieving that first Thanksgiving about her being gone.

Lindsey, I Miss You by Jim Alexander
11-25-2003

Lindsey, I miss you
More than you will know
Each step, each word, each smile
Made my heart glow

Most of all the fun
We had with you around
Cruising on the lake
Or driving around town

Going out to eat
Just isn't any fun
Without you there
Eating more than a ton

Most of all the hugs
And kissing you good-night
Is what I miss the most
They made everything right

Sleep was no problem
Meds weren't that bad
I'd do it for fifty more years
To repeat what we had

Chapter Eighteen

I can't bring you back
But sure do wish I could
Go back several years
And relive our trips for seafood

The joy of Christmas
Just cannot be the same
Without seeing your presents
And hearing them call your name

I could just grieve forever
But God took care of that
He's going to take me too
To see my Lindsey cat

My little buttercup
Has the sweetest smile
My little buttercup
Won't you stay a while?

You and I were meant
For a bicycle built for two
My little buttercup
I love you!

Acknowledgments

My sincere love and gratitude go to my wife and two sons who continue to stand by me through everything. I express great appreciation to Katie Parker, my editor, and to Dr. Elman Frantz, who wrote the foreword. To God and Jesus Christ I owe everything.

About the Author

Jim Alexander is a first-time writer who was inspired to write about his daughter's life. He grew up in the western 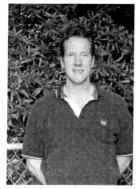 North Carolina foothills where he developed a strong sense of humor and a love of the outdoors, sports, and playing musical instruments, which he enjoys today. He was educated as an industrial engineer and has been involved in managing the development of new products for the last twenty years.

Jim is very involved in working with his two sons in scouting, school, outdoor, and church-related activities. He and his wife and children continue family activities together, especially soccer tournaments and water- and snow-skiing.